# PRAISE FOR
## *THE THRIVING DOCTOR*

*The Thriving Doctor* is a must read for any aspiring doctor, doctor, or anyone who interacts with doctors. As a mid-career doctor, I wish I had this book earlier. It explains so eloquently the numerous factors that lead to doctor burnout, and the necessary internal work required to be able to fully show up to do the important work of doctoring. Beyond prose, this book provides helpful exercises to drive reflection and change. It does not blame the victim, rather it addresses the systemic issues in healthcare. This book provides a pragmatic and wholehearted approach to staying as well as possible in our unwell system.

*Andrea Austin, MD, FACEP, FAAEM, CHSE*
*GSACEP Immediate Past President*

I have really enjoyed the opportunity to read *The Thriving Doctor*. I could hear Sharee's voice talking about concepts that have been part of my personal development, experienced while coaching with her. It was a delight. I am going back to many parts to linger over the descriptions.

For me, Sharee really captured the struggle as well as the magic–the privilege–of being a doctor. Her insight into the tensions that exist, the humanity of being a doctor, and the load that we carry as a result gives her work a credibility that resonates.

The scientist in me is reassured by the evidence she provides. The medical stories are ones to which I can relate. I appreciated the summaries that appeared regularly. The activities and questions challenged me to reflect.

My experience working with Sharee is changing my practice as a doctor and as a woman. My family have noticed that I am less reactive, calmer. I am learning to manage my 'energy spend' on my terms. I have a developing vocabulary that includes words like agency, intention, and values. Now my language is around living into my values and bringing my authentic self with kindness and courage, using my voice.

*Dr Sarah Wilmot, GP Anaesthetist*

My medical degree and specialist training gave me the practical skills I needed to be an excellent doctor. However, I was not well equipped to understand the multiple interpersonal relationships that exist within the health care system that so often wear down and burn out junior and senior medical staff.

Thank you for writing *The Thriving Doctor*. It provides insight and techniques for all doctors to understand the systems we work within and provides the much needed tools to develop our leadership and interpersonal skills. It also reminds us to lean into our vulnerability and humility, which were the very things that attracted us into medicine in the first place.

This book helps us be the doctors we want to be and our patients need us to be.

*Dr Edwina Coghlan, Obstetrician & Gynaecologist, Teacher and Mentor*


*The Thriving Doctor* is a call to arms.

It asks us as doctors to consider who we fundamentally are, and how we can make best use of our *best selves* in the service of our patients and communities. Sharee deftly and clearly implores us to see that we can't hide our struggles from others -our fatigue, burnout and cynicism, and living distant from our values impairs us and damages our patients. It's time for that to stop. No job is worth us dying for. No single doctor's life needs to be the kind of battleground it's become for so many of us.

This book is more than just a rationale for self-care. It is a clear guide with strategies we can use for introspection, reflexivity and action. It should be part of every medical student's required reading. I wish I'd known the powerful value of building skills in mindfulness, emotional intelligence and self-awareness when I'd started my own medical journey.

Sharee's own experiences, and the experiences of caring for doctors through coaching, shine a powerful light into our profession from the outside and give hope that we can each learn to build more sustainability into our working lives as well as take better care of our colleagues. Our best imagined future MUST be one where both doctors and patients can flourish, and Sharee invites us to try new strategies that have been absent from medical education and culture for far too long.

*Dr Elisabeth Wearne, GP and Medical Educator*

Sharee's passion for wellness, for those working in an industry that enables the rest of us to be well, jumps off every page of this comprehensive text. Packed with evidence based, real life examples and practical activities, this is a book that every medical practitioner should have close by. If you live with, or care deeply about a medical practitioner, this book is also for you, as it will deepen your understanding of their reality and give you some great ideas as to how you may provide support to those you love.

*Jane Porter, MCC GAICD*


*The Thriving Doctor* is a gift to doctors everywhere, whether they are already thriving in their life or they are struggling with burnout. This is more than a book on thriving — it is a complete how-to guide for self-awareness and mindset mastery. In language that is approachable and easy to read, without unnecessary academic minutiae, Sharee's writing respects the time pressures we are all under in healthcare.

Sharee makes a powerful case for devoting energy to developing self-awareness, and providing the tools to develop that life-changing skill. *The Thriving Doctor* is written from Sharee's vast real-world experience with doctors in every stage of their career and along the stress-well-being spectrum. She writes with a deep and palpable sense of compassion and care for doctors.

There is practical wisdom here that we never got as medical students or at any time during our career. I enjoyed the introduction to the power of coaching for physicians, many of whom may be resistant or uncertain. The section on the culture of medicine and the roots of imposter syndrome during medical training spoke to me directly. Emotional intelligence was covered beautifully. I especially appreciated the brief case studies that serve as real-world examples.

This book and the practices it contains will make me a more effective doctor, colleague, and leader. I'm also certain any physician taking the time to work through this book will reap benefits outside of healthcare, as spouses, parents, and friends.

Brava!!!!

*Jonathan Fisher, MD FACC Cardiologist,*
*Organizational Well-Being & Resiliency Leader*

I would highly recommend this book to all doctors, and to medical students, especially those in their final year. Plain and simple, the book is an engaging read with lots of "aha" moments. *The Thriving Doctor* connects the reader to the stories of doctors who have encountered and effectively managed issues in the clinical workplace. The book provides insights into the processes underpinning coaching. It shows the reader the tried and trusted steps to build skills for more effective and satisfying engagement with the whole clinical workplace.

This book also works as a manual to build adaptive behaviours step by step to move from surviving or enduring to flourishing and thriving. That this is not an easy task is acknowledged, the book is grounded in reality. Sharee highlights that thriving does not mean an absence of distress. Like any skill, engagement and practice is key. When the focus shifts to effectively prioritise self, it will feel right!

*Associate Professor Catherine Haigh,*
*Director, Monash Rural Health Gippsland*

*The Thriving Doctor* has amazing depth, so much so that it is not possible to absorb all in one read. It is relevant to both medical and non-medical practitioners, with valuable pearls that challenge our way of thinking. Previously assumed terms are redefined into relevant and useful practical solutions to the challenges our modern day workforce, and life, presents.

Sharee structures her book in a logical sequence, with practical 'to do' tasks that allow us to pause and reflect, and indeed self-discover. This book complements the workshops and courses run by Sharee and allows us to explore these concepts in further depth, almost like a core textbook and reference.

I would urge all junior doctors to read this to pick up a few learning points. It will also be worth revisiting later, as new challenges in your career or new situations arise or new levels of maturity are reached. I know if I had discovered this earlier I would have avoided a fair amount of hurt and distress, and be much further along the path to thriving.

*Dr Antony Wong, GP Anaesthetist*

This book doesn't need a critique or a review. It's complete. It's a gift to our profession, one for every medical student and doctor, junior and senior.
First Sharee articulated the way that I feel.
Then she gave me permission to acknowledge my feelings.
She made me feel valued. She made me realise that I mattered.
Sharee encouraged me to confront my emotions, and to challenge my existing paradigm, and told me that was ok.
  ...and then she gave me the tools with which to make a change.

*Dr Vijay Roach, Obstetrician and Gynaecologist, Past President RANZCOG*


I am so grateful for Sharee and the work she does. Sharee's teaching is another curriculum, too often not easily accessible and vital for all doctors' professional development. Her teachings and practical advice can salvage careers and save lives.

*Dr Bree Wyeth, Psychiatrist*


An evidenced based guidebook for preventing or recovering from burnout to leading an intentional and meaningful life.
  This is a book that we can all benefit from, starting from where we are right now, to be more effective as doctors and more engaged with life. A recommended read for all doctors, I'll be giving it to all of my colleagues.
  Thank you Sharee for writing this book. Your clear writing, the evidence based content, and practical exercises have challenged and supported me to evolve how I think about my identity as a doctor. I feel better equipped to balance this with my other needs to live a meaningful and thriving life.

*Dr Louise Sterling, GP and Practice Owner*


Sharee is an extraordinary human being, and a kind and compassionate coach. Over the many years we've worked together on patient centred care, communication, and patient safety, Sharee has made connections between concepts, people, and communities where it was most needed.

One of Sharee's greatest strengths is in how well she listens to our stories. It is this attention that has enabled her to truly capture the essence of other people's lived experiences, in particular in a medical context. I have seen the skill with which she facilitates panels in person, and she has carried this sensitivity and perception into her writing of this book. This clarity of thought is why she is so perfectly qualified to work with Doctors to find their own balance.

With gentle expertise she has woven these lessons into a wise and enduring resource that will change the lives of doctors everywhere. It is strengthened by beautiful illustrations that showcase the intersection between arts and medicine. Through challenging and joyful examples, Sharee continues to advocate for doctors to advocate for themselves.

*Prof Catherine Crock AM, Founder, Hush Foundation*

# ACKNOWLEDGEMENT

I would like to respectfully acknowledge the First Nation people of Country throughout Australia, especially the traditional owners of the land where I live and wrote this book, the Gunaikurnai people.

I acknowledge the cultural and spiritual connection that Aboriginal and Torres Strait Islander peoples have with the land and sea. I remain committed to listening, learning, growing, and being together on what was, and always will be, Aboriginal land that has never been ceded.

First published in 2021 by Hambone Publishing
Melbourne, Australia

Illustrations by Glenn Finlay
Edited by Mish Phillips, Danielle Upshall and Emily Stephenson
Interior Design by David W. Edelstein
Cover design by Andrea Hall, Gio Abarquez, Russell Caras and Daniela Florez
Cover photo of Sharee by Lisa Baker

For information about this title, contact:
Sharee Johnson
sharee@skjconsulting.com.au
www.coachingfordoctors.net.au

ISBN 978-1-922357-26-7 (paperback)
ISBN 978-1-922357-27-4 (eBook)
ISBN 978-1-922357-33-5 (audiobook)

*Remembering Tim*

*To my awesome teachers Will, Ella and Tess*

*and*

*Dedicated to every doctor, thank you*

# The Thriving Doctor

**Sharee Johnson**
Illustrated by Glenn Finlay

# GRATITUDE

In my roles as psychologist, coach, and meditation teacher, I do a lot of listening to what is said and what is unsaid. There is often a lot of emotion present when I sit with another person, a doctor. In my practice and in this book, I have tried to bear testimony to what I see and hear from doctors, to hold safe space for you to explore your experiences, and to offer practical psychological responses that you can use in your day-to-day life to maintain your wellbeing and prevent burnout in the face of many wicked challenges.

To support, encourage, and occasionally guide you while you experiment and learn is one of my life's privileges. I have learnt so much from every doctor I have sat with. I am humbled by your commitment to your endlessly challenging work, your willing service to our community, and the trust you have offered me. Thank you doctors for taking care of us.

Before I worked with doctors, I worked with people from all walks of life as a therapist and in many other roles. My deep gratitude to everyone who has ever consulted me as client, colleague, or student participant, your trust and partnership over the past 30 years have allowed me to learn how to take psychological theory and research into real living. Thank you for all the lived wisdom you have shared with me. Remember, you are already more than you think you are.

A deep bow of gratitude and thanks to my mentors and coaches over the years: Elizabeth Roylance, Kerry Brydon, Angela Forbes, Jeanette Gibson, Debra Smith, Nick Thurbon, Uli Kimler, Nick Petrucco, Justine Anderson, Pam Newton, Rasmus Hougaard, Gillian Coutes, Mike Allen,

Lindel Greggory, Sabina Vitacca, Jo Klap, Fuyuko Toyota, Karen Soltes, Vicki Crabb, Elisabeth Wearne, Catherine Crock, Lucy Mayes, Vijay Roach, John Matthews, Jane Porter and Andrew Green. And all my colleagues along the way who have been willing to dig deep into life with me, sometimes digging around in a lot of dirt to find a tiny speck of gold. Thank you for your patience and respect, your willingness to share and, most of all, your belief in me. Thank you also to those who may not realise how key their mentorship from afar has been in my development: Ian Gawler, Munjed Al Muderis, Richard Miller, Mehrdad Nikfarjam and David Clutterbuck.

I cannot really remember a time in my life without books. I often joke I will die drowning in them. Books have provided me with adventure, challenge, solace, and a continuous stream of learning. This book stands on the shoulders of giants in psychology, neuroscience, leadership coaching, philosophy, and spirituality. Thank you to all the authors and researchers who have asked what seemed like impossible questions and found ways for us to understand them, progressing our understanding of the human condition.

This book would not have happened without Kelly Irving and the incredible community of authors she brings together. Thank you, Kelly, for reminding me that writing is thinking and for being willing to walk through all the early iterations of that thinking with me. Thank you to everyone in the expert author community for inspiring and encouraging me to keep writing.

To everyone at Hambone Publishing, especially editors Michelle Phillips, Danielle Upshall, and Emily Stephenson, who have helped craft what is mostly a private world of coaching in practice, into an accessible resource. Thank you to David Edelstein for his design work, making the book easy to navigate. And to publishing master Ben Phillips, for taking such good care of me and *The Thriving Doctor* as it enters the world.

To my friend Glenn Finlay for keeping art in our lives, always. Working on this book with you has been such a treat. You have added so much humanity and warmth to the story telling of *The Thriving Doctor* with your fabulous drawings. Thank you, Glenn.

Thank you to the early readers of this manuscript: Elisabeth Wearne,

Joel Fanning, Elise Ly, Rachel Fanning, Nicola Finlay, Rachel Patton, Cath Crock, Cathy Haigh, Lucy Mayes, Tanya Preston, Ziena Al-Obaidi, Sharon Ray, Andrea Hall, Antony Wong, Iris Tung, Robert Anderson, Chris Sellers, Sarah Bass, Adrian Jobson, Vijay Roach, Jane Porter, Bree Wyeth, Jonathan Fisher, Andrea Austin, Edwina Coghlan, Louise Sterling and Sarah Wilmot. Your feedback has made anything I could write so much better.

Thank you to Andrea Hall and Linda Hunt for keeping Coaching for Doctors ticking, from the genesis of early community events in 2014, to what is now a thriving practice serving hundreds of doctors. Andrea, you have kept me sane during the writing of this book; thank you for your organisational expertise, patience, enthusiasm, design ideas, and endless encouragement.

Thank you to Cameron Roberts, Tiffany Jao, and Ethan Brown, who helped me rise to the challenge that was 2020. Tika Reeves, thank you for keeping things moving in 2021. You have all embraced the vision of driving a healthier healthcare system by taking better care of doctors with passion and commitment, and for that I am grateful. Moving mountains is much more fun with company.

To my psychologist colleagues, the coaching community, the meditation teacher community, everyone at Pancare and to the healthcare movement communities I am a part of — Gathering of Kindness, Compassion Revolution, Ending Physician Burnout, and our own Recalibrate Alumni community — keep going! Belonging is central to wellbeing; I know that my wellbeing is enhanced by each of these communities, and I commend their work to everyone. They can help you put your wellbeing first. Together we can all be better and feel better; it takes a village to stay well, and it's forever work. Together we can transform healthcare.

Anything I have achieved has happened because of the secure, loving family I have been blessed to live in. Thank you, Mum and Dad; you set me up to *give it a go*, whatever *it* might be in any given moment, decades ago. Rachel, Dean and Joel, I feel so lucky to share the same orbit with you three; thank you for reading, advising, and talking straight. To Will, Ella and Tess, you three are the stars that light my sky. Thank you for being patient these past two years especially, when work has taken over. It has been a silver lining of the COVID lockdowns to have had extra time with you three. I love you always.

My first village also includes the rest of the Fanning-Oliver clan, especially Noel, Nicki and Elise, who have helped take such good care of us these past 10 years. Thank you to the Johnson-Boyd clan, especially Libby, Johnny, Paul, Rachel, Tony and Nat, for keeping us close. Libby, Paul and Rachel, your ability to anticipate what we need and simply show up is something to behold; thank you. Big tight hugs to our extra family Nicola, Glenn, Tom, and Kate for loving us, taking care of us, and teaching us so many things. To Jo and Chris Jones who have looked out for us and made us laugh. To my beautiful sisterhood, especially Nicola Finlay, Naomi Hatwell, Tanya Preston, Jane Cameron, Nikki Smith, Pam Newton and Donna Rowand, thank you for being my trusty sounding boards. Thank you to Paul Johnson, Andrew Cameron, Nick Cox, Duncan Smith, Mick Hatwell, and Chris Rowand, my go-to guys. Thank you all for the constant acceptance and love you have given me. Thank you to all my glorious friends, I can't wait to hug you again; you make my life rich. I have so much to savour and be grateful for.

And of course, to Tim who trusted me and is still my guiding light.

Choose your attitude and take action; you have but one precious life. May you all be well! XS

# AUTHOR'S NOTE

A note on client confidentiality: I have changed names and all identifying particulars to preserve the anonymity of those doctors who trust me as their coach. Where I have written about some part of their story, I have sought their permission, and all have agreed to share their experience in the interests of better wellbeing and care for doctors.

# CONTENTS

**Thriving:** adjective

*Prosperous and growing; flourishing* (Oxford)

*Someone or something that is doing well
and is successful, healthy, or strong* (Collins)

# INTRODUCTION

The experienced medical director sitting opposite me in coaching said: "You were the first person to ever ask me: – *what do you want?*"

He went on to describe the profound impact this simple question had had on him. These four words had given him permission to discover, to imagine, to believe that he could meet some of his own needs once he knew what they were.

These four words had freed him from the straight jacket the culture of medicine had bound him in for 25 years and ultimately allowed him to practise medicine with renewed energy and focus. He felt happier, stronger, and was enjoying his family and his work more than he had for two decades.

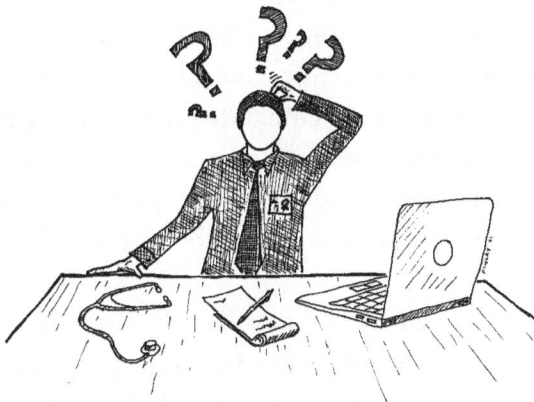

## PATIENTS WILL BENEFIT TOO

I understand that in your role as doctor you are committed to patient safety and patient health. You are possibly only interested in reading books that impact positively on patient care. On this front the research is very clear. **Well doctors are better doctors, and they help their patients achieve better health outcomes.**

The Institute of Medicine described the primary determinants of healthcare quality in 2001; one of which was patient-centred care. They described this as "Healthcare that establishes a partnership among practitioners, patients and their families". Further to this, they concluded that patient-centred care is nothing less than a "Quality and business imperative", and that "In general, **most patients feel confident** that they will receive **competent technical care** when they enter a hospital or healthcare centre". Beyond that, "**What matters most** to them is being **treated with kindness, compassion and dignity**".

A doctor who builds positive relationships with their patients is perceived by them as more empathic and more compassionate. These patients continue with their treatment more consistently and for longer duration. Not surprisingly they have better health outcomes including faster recovery rates and better immune response.

The healing power of positive interactions has been well documented, and often forgotten in the measurement of success in healthcare. For example, Rakel et al (2009 and 2011) compared recovery time and immune responses of three groups of patients with upper respiratory tract infections. Immune response was most vigorous and recovery time shortest in patients with empathic physicians. Recovery time was longest for the group with doctors who lacked empathy – longer than those who saw no doctor at all! Rakel and team concluded that empathy in the therapeutic encounter resulted in faster recovery times for flu patients.

The science of medicine is data-driven, humans may not be. Doctors are humans first; emotional beings like their patients, being asked to ignore the art of medicine to their own and their patients' detriment.

> **Raising your capacity to care for yourself improves patient health outcomes, patient experience and patient safety.**

As you prioritise taking better care of yourself, you have greater capacity to be empathic, compassionate and patient centred. As you raise the care of your patients by being well yourself and raising your skills, you can build confidence, trust and respect in yourself, and others too will have more confidence, trust and respect in you.

Your state of health and wellbeing must come first. All other health-care goals ride on this. Only when you have the skills to take care of yourself effectively can you truly take care of anyone else properly.

## YOU CAN MAKE A DIFFERENCE IN YOUR OWN MEDICAL LIFE

There is a great deal every individual doctor can do to improve their own experience at work in the healthcare system and in medicine – for both themselves and their patients. To do so you need to engage your own agency, the same agency you used to get into medicine in the first place.

> **Personal agency is a sense of control over your own actions and the consequences.**

When you do exercise your personal agency, you bring your influence to bear on what you can control in your own life. Exercising control over your thoughts, motivation, and actions, you remember and hold dearly the belief that you can make decisions and enact them for your own benefit. In this empowered state you are also more likely to make a difference for those around you.

Surgeon and former CEO of Keiser Permanente Dr Robert Pearl says in his book *Uncaring (2021)* that medicine has taught doctors how to cure people, but it has not done such a good job of teaching you how to *care* for them. He is pointing to the science of medicine being more valued than the art of medicine. Whether you agree with Dr Pearl or not, I think we can take it a step further and recognise that medicine has not done a good job of teaching *you how to care for yourself* in the face of the work you do.

Did anyone actively teach you how to maintain your health and wellbeing so that you could be the best doctor you can be? So that you can continue performing your work at your best for the long term in the face of so much human suffering?

Medicine has more likely actively trained you to look after others first and by implication to neglect your own wellbeing. Many of the structures, systems and much of the culture of medicine has even rewarded you for neglecting your own wellbeing. Although it was probably not any individual's intention, this has had the impact of creating risk for patients and for providers.

> **This book is about what you can do as a doctor beyond technical clinical skill to be a safe, trusted, high-performing doctor who achieves career longevity, satisfaction and wellbeing as you go.**

Your technical clinical skills are not necessarily going to help you cope with fatigue, unsuccessful patient treatments, giving bad news to patients, sleep deprivation, bullying, trauma, or self-doubt. **Your non-clinical skills are essential to delivering the best medical care.** Underdeveloped, they limit your success with patients and reduce your wellbeing, now and over the course of your medical career. To be the best doctor you can be, you must also pay attention to developing your interpersonal skills and your internal regulation skills (intrapersonal). Who knows, you may even come to see these skills as essential clinical skills!

> **Take care of yourself first, that is within your control.**

## BECOMING AN AGENT OF CHANGE IN YOUR OWN LIFE

> **Prevention is better than a cure.**

I hope to help you activate yourself to build the skills you need for a joyful, fulfilling, satisfying life in medicine. This book is **not** focused on what to do *after* you have burned out, it is about how to break that pattern. This book does not promise you more happiness, though according to the doctors I have worked with it's a likely by-product. **This book is about prevention, personal agency, empowerment, finding and keeping your balance, and human connection.** In these pages, you will reconnect with the agency you have called on to get this far in your medical career. These skills can help you thrive and flourish.

You will learn the skills you need to be able to take charge of yourself, building on them to:

- perform your work at a high level
- lead others effectively and warmly
- maintain your wellbeing throughout a long-term medical career
- achieve more work-life balance.

When you do, when you are flourishing, everyone else around you will reap the benefits too and the systems will change, because the systems are made up of people. Medicine is a human construct, built and delivered by humans for humans.

> **Well, effective, empowered people respond to and create different systems to those who are burned out, disappointed and ill-equipped.**

## SELF-CARE IS ESSENTIAL FOR YOU TO MAINTAIN YOUR MEDICAL CAREER

Investing in your self-care skills (intrapersonal) – mindfulness, compassion, emotional intelligence – and your relationship skills (interpersonal) – communication, collaboration, leadership – will help you become a better doctor with a more sustainable career that includes better patient outcomes, a better reputation and more satisfaction.

> Self-care requires your consistent effort, on purpose every day.

Self-care is less about bubble baths and going for a run (though these are useful), and more about **what's truly deeply important to you**. The key question then really is:

1. Do you think taking care of your physical and psychological health is *worth your effort?*

If you answered yes, we must ask another question:

2. Are you *willing* to make that effort in the service of your own goals including your wellbeing?

It's the elephant in the room for most doctors, always putting the patient first and leaving yourself for later. You've probably been saying "Look after yourself first" to patients for years. Remember that single parent you told to take care of herself so she could take better care of her kids? Or that person with diabetes who you talked to about making small efforts every day to stay well?

Are you walking your talk in your own life?

Do you know how to create the life conditions that will see you thrive or has medicine (the system) clouded your view?

How do you rate your wellbeing right now out of 10?

Honestly, how are you doing at looking after yourself?

## A COACH'S LENS

I work as a specialist psychologist coach. My clients are doctors. There is one message I would love doctors to take to heart, to really embed in their lives:

> **Make looking after yourself first your absolute priority. Then you will be a better, more fulfilled doctor who can thrive in a long-term sustainable medical career.**

I help doctors develop the skills they need to be more effective in terms of performance, leadership and wellbeing. This allows them to continue their medical careers long term with joy, satisfaction and life balance. Coaching is an evidence based, forward facing, achievement focused process. Our work is measured as successful by the doctors when their skilful actions and increasing internal capacity result in a more fulfilling, balanced life.

Coaching helps doctors to focus on thinking clearly, understanding what hinders and helps them, and activating their own energy in the service of their values and goals. It's a confidential, proactive process that seeks to understand and activate the doctor (coachee) in line with *their* purpose. Skills, insight, clarity, and action are the tools we use.

Professionally, my understanding of the world comes from working as a psychologist for nearly 30 years. As a non-doctor, I have not been indoctrinated by medicine; I am not a part of the medical hierarchy and not bound by the same cultural rules and norms. **This is important because it means I ask different questions of the doctors I work with than I would if I was a fish swimming in the same water.** I do not accept the same things, I do not take the same things for granted as you do, and I have not been inculcated. I look at medicine with fresh eyes and curiosity.

> Medical education is largely blind to intra- and interpersonal
> skills, describing them as non-clinical and disregarding
> them for at least a century.

Which is why I established Australia's first psychologist coaching practice exclusively for doctors in 2015. Medicine is different to other careers. Doctors from across the country have taught me about their culture and the realities of medicine. Every day they tell me their demoralised stories of poor feedback, failed competencies, rude colleagues, abuses of power and systemic failure. Every day we work to rebuild their confidence, find a values-based way forward and challenge the system.

The work we do at Coaching for Doctors is about personal development and to that extent often involves the deep work of introspection including exploring values and emotions. You can expect to talk a lot about your intention, values and goals, both known and emerging, through the process of coaching and in this book.

There is no promise or guarantee of an easy road. Yet, with the right skills and a mindset determined to take care of you, we can see you delivering on your intention to work as a doctor for the long term and be well. You are human first, a doctor second.

## WHICH DOCTORS ARE USING COACHING?

There are four broad kinds of responses doctors have to the idea of working with a psychologist coach:

1.  The first group expresses interest, is surprised that such a role exists, and very warmly encourages me, saying many doctors will need coaching. Generally, these doctors see themselves as well and fulfilled by their work. Sometimes they refer their colleagues. Not every doctor needs coaching all the time.

2.  The second group of doctors are having a crisis – disillusioned, burned out, recently having had a serious adverse event with a patient, considering leaving medicine, having failed an important exam, or facing the reality of not being accepted onto a training program. Some of these doctors I refer to counselling for trauma and grief. Some start coaching with me to resolve their options, clarify their values and goals and make changes in their life.

3.  The third group have heard about coaching and recognise it as a way to build their skills and progress their careers. These doctors have noticed that medical training has not given them everything they need to be truly effective. They recognise that coaching is a process that has successfully helped many other professionals lift their performance and meet their goals. They are ready and willing to commit to doing the work of personal development that underpins their professional development. These doctors have noticed a skills gap between where they are and where they want to be. Often, they are moving into a leadership role, or they might have had some feedback that they don't know how to respond to, like … *you need to be more empathic.* This group is also proactively trying to create more work-life balance.

4.  There is possibly a fourth polite group who don't understand how a non-doctor has anything to offer, but they keep it to themselves!

> Whatever you think about working with a coach, I want you to know that 100% of the doctors I have met agree that the way they were trained did not give them all the skills they needed to be a truly effective doctor.

## WHAT SKILLS NEED DEVELOPING?

I asked a sample of Australian doctors from various specialties what they thought a psychologist coach could help doctors learn that might help them be more effective in their work. Surprisingly, they all said versions of doctors *do not know themselves*.

They talked about three key themes:

1. Why do so many doctors end up with a **mental health** issue when they know about mental health?
2. The culture of **perfectionism and the inherent competition** in medicine is damaging
3. That all doctors are under **pressure especially regarding time**, so they don't invest in themselves. Self-care always has to wait, especially in the early years, which means doctors live with a whole lot of bad habits and unhelpful thinking.

## PUT YOURSELF FIRST — A NEW PARADIGM

This simple idea is not easy for any doctor working in our complex health-care system to deliver when they have been raised on an ethos of *patient first*. This book is an invitation to shift your thinking a bit. This is not some flight of fancy, the skills and ideas in these pages have been tried and tested by your doctor colleagues over several years.

> The doctors I work with consistently tell me these skills have helped them become better doctors and more fulfilled people.

Developing their intra- and interpersonal skills has made a big difference in their lives, including in their medical work. Consistently applying the skills and strategies described in these pages can help you change your medical life, benefiting you and your patients, helping you achieve personally and professionally. These are the skills adults need to thrive.

Developing these skills will help you flourish and result in better healthcare for your patients, but don't do it for them! Do it for yourself and your own family. If you do, you can be confident your patients and colleagues will also benefit. When you are thriving, it's contagious, the impact ripples out widely.

> **If you take one message away from this book, I hope it is to invest in yourself.**

Make time for you and make it your absolute number one priority. Schedule it in your diary as if your life and the lives of your patients depend on it – because they do. No one else can do it for you, and no one will. Investing in yourself can give you:

- clarity of mind
- emotional stability
- a clear sense of purpose
- career longevity
- agency at work
- more energy and joy
- better relationships
- more work-life balance.

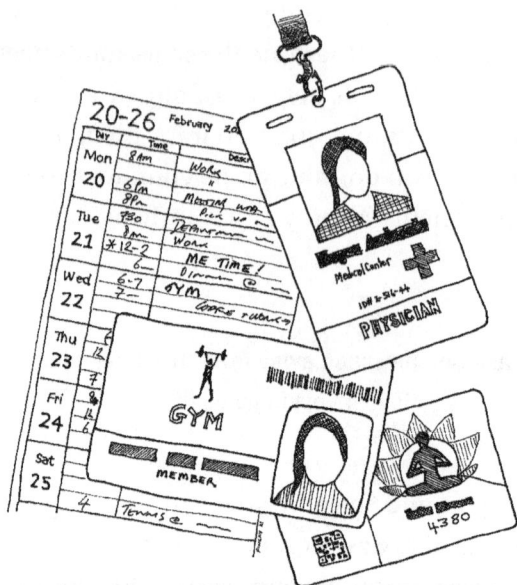

Work-life balance isn't a mystery, even in medicine. It's a series of habits that become routine. It's a skill set that you practise like with any other skill you want to develop. It's a conscious effort that exercises your personal agency, empowering you to live how *you* choose rather than the system making you into a victim. You have used your personal agency to get this far, I'm inviting you to use it again to design the life you want even while you work in healthcare.

To do so, you need to know what it is you want for your life. Imagine being clear about what gives your life meaning, being purposeful in your actions and clear of mind. Imagine achieving the right work-life balance for you and your family, enjoying your work, having strong trusting relationships with your colleagues and building a medical practice that is sustainable.

> **This book is about the tools you need to look after yourself. When you use them consistently and skilfully you will be well and more effective. You will be much more able to deliver optimal care to your patients.**

## WHY READ THIS BOOK / HOW TO USE THIS BOOK

I get that you are time poor and reading a book about improving your performance and wellbeing might seem like a luxury. I promise, it's a short-term pain for a long-term gain. You, your family, your patients, their families, and your colleagues will benefit from your decision to take action.

Make a commitment to yourself today and make one change in your life in service of a better life. Give yourself 45 minutes and read one chapter.

You picked up this book for a reason, what did you hope to find? What is it that you need? Are you ready to take one small step towards a better medical life? Step wisely into your own power with humility and readiness to learn.

> **Think of learning these non-clinical skills like superannuation, the sooner you invest in them the greater return you, your patients and your family will get.**

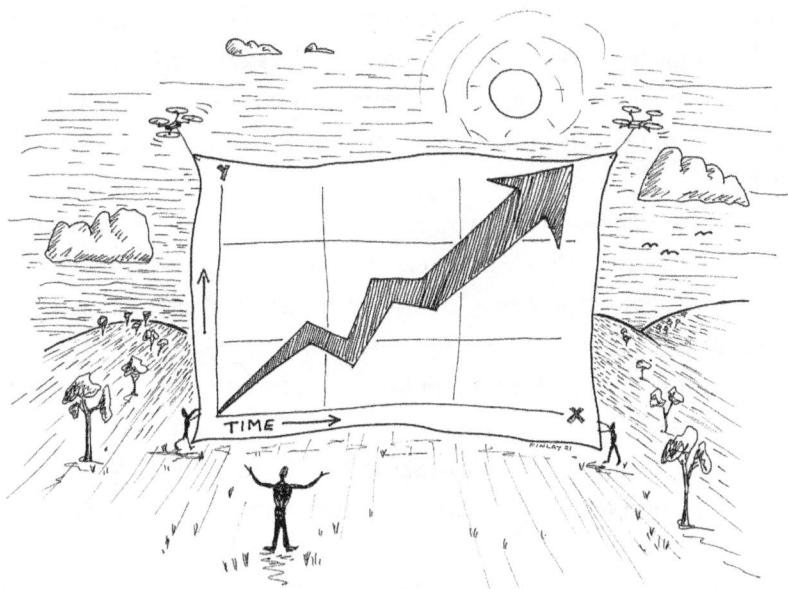

You can use the tools and the tested theoretical frameworks from neuroscience and positive psychology in this book to start this work yourself. You'll do better with a coach beside you. Intelligent, capable doctors like to think they can solve every problem, ideally on their own. The problem is, you're too busy solving everyone else's problems to ever tend properly to your own! When you give yourself a coach, you gain an external perspective and the accountability you need to look after your own challenges, making you more effective personally and professionally.

This book is divided into two parts.

Part one, **Chapters 1 and 2**, focuses on why *you* are the key to your future. It's not surprising that working as a doctor comes with risk. In 2021 it's well known in the doctor community that burnout, depression, and suicide rates are high. The problems of healthcare draw on your energy as a doctor constantly.

Yet everything exists within a context. Understanding your context is important because it affects what you think of as possible, how you feel and behave. The reverse is also true of course. Your internal environment – how you think and feel – can also affect your external environment.

When we understand the context you work in that creates your thinking and emotions, then we can really understand what will help you flourish. Instead of reacting to your environment, you can build a mature inner scaffold, helping you to respond more effectively and allowing you to thrive.

Part two, **Chapters 3 through 9**, focuses on *how* to activate your agency and thrive. These chapters are about empowering you. Each chapter includes suggestions for how you can start practising the skills discussed and implementing them in your day-to-day life to help you thrive. Habit change is best made one step at a time in tiny incremental doses. Behaviour that you can repeat often is the best way to help your plastic brain reshape in the direction you want to go. For example, 5 minutes of meditation every day is more effective than 30 minutes once a week.

There is a logical order to the chapters in part two that follows the established pattern of our group programs, which doctors have codesigned with me over the years. However, you can read any chapter on its own and start anywhere your interest takes you.

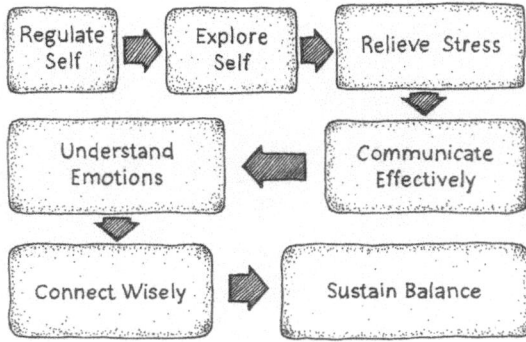

Regulate Self → Explore Self → Relieve Stress

Understand Emotions ← Communicate Effectively

Connect Wisely → Sustain Balance

Don't wait for a crisis before you commit to putting yourself first.

There will be plenty of opportunities to reflect as you work your way through this book. If you have a journal, you might like to keep it nearby. If you don't already have a practice of reflective writing, you might like to start as you read this book. You can amplify the impact of your learning when you write about it and when you talk about it with others. These practices make the ideas your own as you start to think about how they apply to your real life. There is some truth to the medical maxim 'see one, do one, teach one.' If you want to amplify the impact of these tools in your life, find a coach to help you.

# 1

# THE HARSH REALITY
# OF HEALTHCARE

*"Healthcare is the most difficult,
chaotic and complex industry to manage."*
*— Peter Drucker*

## Sandro's Story

Sandro worked as a psychiatrist in a busy health network. He was committed to working in public health, as he felt that's where his skills were most needed. Although the organisational chart showed three psychiatrists in his department, in the three years he had worked there he had only had one six-month period working with a psychiatrist colleague. The workload was huge, constant, complex, and draining. Many more patients needed inpatient beds than were available. Every day, he and the mental health nurses met with families who were out of their minds with fear about what their psychologically unstable relative would do next, and desperate to escalate the level of care provided to their family member.

Sandro found himself saying, 'Our hands are tied'. Yet this was not the kind of psychiatrist he wanted to be. He thought about going into private practice, he thought about working part time, and as he said to me, he had thought of leaving medicine altogether many times. Every way he looked, Sandro felt vulnerable. The safe space of coaching became his sanity while he processed these thoughts out loud.

*On a daily basis, he asked: 'How can I do the work I feel passionate about, when the system is not set up for me to do that? How can I meet the needs of these most needy of patients?'. He was committed to the work. His heart beat for public healthcare that was accessible to everyone. And yet, it seemed like a hopeless cause.*

Can you relate?

## IT'S THE SYSTEM

There are three things doctors consistently tell me they want in their lives and in their medical practice:

1. **Patient safety.** They want to have confidence that they are a safe practitioner, and they want their patients and their colleagues to know and respect them as a safe practitioner.

2. **To be trusted** to make good decisions. They want to trust themselves and be trusted by others because they have put a lot of effort into being a good doctor.

3. **A better work-life balance**, less stress, and a feeling of fulfilment.

> Most doctors I have met lament "the system" as the thing that thwarts them in their effort to be safe, trustworthy, and achieve more balance in their work.

It is the system they name as the key limiting factor to their success. The *system* generally means the whole of healthcare being complex and unwieldy. And sometimes it means medicine; the way doctors are trained and how they progress in their careers.

Both medicine and the healthcare system have significant problems. Like all complex systems they are continually evolving, but progress is slow. In complex systems, change in one part affects the rest of the system. In large complex systems, it can be hard to identify the impact in real time. Often the way change in one part of the system impacts another part of the system can only be seen in hindsight.

> You signed up to help people, yet the system and culture of medicine means some days you wonder if you can even help yourself.

The healthcare system undermines, sabotages, and counteracts the effort doctors are making in service of their patients, taking away their opportunity to feel satisfied or fulfilled in their work.

While it is true that systemic change is desperately needed in healthcare and medicine, blaming the external environment you train and work in doesn't help you to progress your leadership, performance, or wellbeing in the short- and medium-term.

Systemic and cultural transformation of healthcare won't happen overnight. They can be ignited in any moment though. We have seen plenty of this during the Covid pandemic; telehealth is a good example of how things can progress much quicker than we had previously thought.

> Focus more on your own skills and capacity than on the system. Systemic change can be a by-product of what you do for yourself in your area of healthcare. Start with yourself, lead yourself well.

## DECIDING TO BECOME A DOCTOR

When you decided to go to medical school, you began a journey with inherent risks to your psychological and physical health. You couldn't have begun to understand what that meant back then.

## Reflection

- What did you hope to do and be with your medical degree one day?
- What was your intention back then?
- What has been driving you, what kept you going all this time?
- What has been motivating you?
- What has allowed you to sacrifice so much of your own life and your own wellbeing that you have kept at it through all the challenges?

You knew intellectually you would see broken, bloody, hysterical, and dead people. Of course, knowing it was nothing like being confronted by actual real broken, bloody, hysterical, and dead people. Now that you have some experience with broken, bloody, hysterical people, now that you have broken bad news and sat in the company of death, what keeps you going?

When you were accepted into medicine, it was only the first step in a long line of challenges you have been asked to meet. Five or six years of rigorous written and practical examinations followed by the confusing and competitive process of seeking a place on a training program where demand outstrips supply. Competing with your friends and colleagues for jobs and training places, while also supporting each other at the bottom of the pecking order, brings its own complexity. You may have been working as an unaccredited doctor or a registrar for what feels like an eternity.

To become an independent specialist doctor means giving up a social life, being tested and assessed about everything, year after year climbing a steep hierarchy. After you fellow, you continue to work hard to maintain your colleagues' esteem, your referral base, the safety of your patients. Becoming a doctor is a day-by-day process of repeated exposure to hardship – your own and other people's.

> Medicine requires your ongoing high performance and energy throughout your career, it never really ends.

## THE ART AND SCIENCE OF MEDICINE

Science and technology have advanced medicine exponentially. Through rigorous scientific method, medicine has discovered antibiotics, the impact of hand hygiene, dialysis, the EEG, pacemaker, MRI, the insulin pump, and the cochlear implant. It is easy to get excited by these advances and want to focus on them. Perhaps the sheer amount of clinical and technical information you need to wrap your mind around leaves little room for finessing other, non-clinical skills.

For a century or so, medicine has tilted more and more toward science. This book is not about the emancipation of science or clinical skill. It is about understanding that the other skills – those you might think of as soft skills or non-clinical skills – are therapeutic and also advance medicine. You can be a better doctor for your own fulfilment and for the patient's health when you also pay attention to the art of medicine, which includes managing emotions, building good relationships, and communicating effectively.

> Interpersonal skills and internal management skills will complement and enhance your clinical skills more than you realise if you have never paid much attention to them.

There have been good reasons for medicine to focus on science and to suppress emotions. You are confronted multiple times a day with human suffering. During times of war, famine and depression, this human suffering has been immeasurable. Traditionally, medicine has kept a lid on this reality by teaching doctors implicitly and explicitly to keep their emotions suppressed.

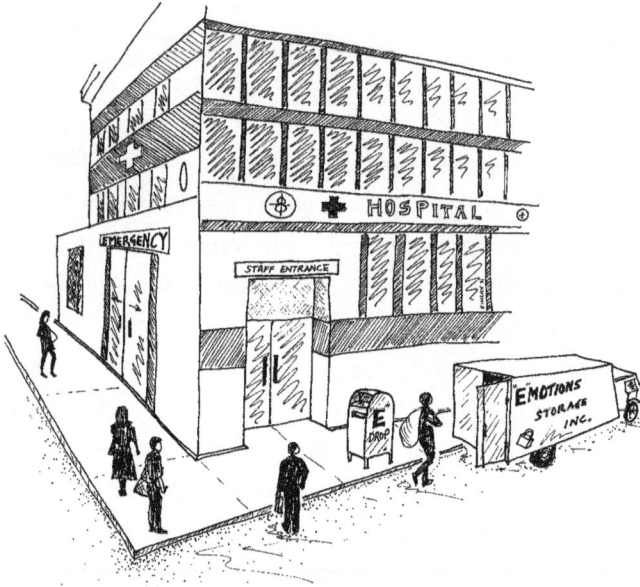

## STOICISM AND RESILIENCE

Decades of burying and ignoring emotions has created a medical culture that values and promotes the scientific method, and stoicism in doctors. In recent times, healthcare has confused stoicism with resilience – they are not the same. Modern stoicism, according to the Oxford Dictionary, is "The endurance of pain or hardship without the display of feelings and without complaint". According to organisational psychologist, Kathryn McEwan, who developed the Resilience at Work assessment tool, resilience is an ability to manage stress, to learn and adapt, integrating this new learning as you go forward. There is no exclusion of emotion required for resilience. Resilience is more concerned with learning and adapting, and stoicism is more about carrying on no matter what.

> As you trained to be a good doctor, you learnt to disconnect emotionally from the people around you so you could compete and be objective. In doing so, you lost some of your potential healing capacity and along with it some of your potential joy.

The process and strategy of ignoring interpersonal connection and intrapersonal experience hasn't worked for many patients, doctors, or for either group's families. Broadly speaking, there are two main reasons for this failure. The first is that emotions are present in everything we think and do. The second is that we are social animals, relying on human connection to survive, especially when we are sick and vulnerable. We are hardwired for connection. Our emotions are critical for bonding; they evolved as a species survival strategy. We are not designed for total independence and objectivity.

> **The culture of medicine values stoicism, competition, and perfectionism.**

This medical culture of modern stoicism is sometimes described as the hidden curriculum of medicine. It includes being willing to work long hours, to always put the patient first, to never say you cannot cope (for fear of others deeming you not up to the job or weak), and to avoid saying that you don't know, or you need help, at all costs. This culture fosters the internal voice of imposter syndrome.

After being indoctrinated into this skewed culture for two or three years at medical school learning how to be a clinical, evidence-based doctor, you started seeing real patients with your supervisors. At the same time, you may have begun to wonder whether you *really have what it takes to be a doctor.*

As a young doctor it may have felt like there was just not enough cognitive space to think about intra- and interpersonal skills. Your inner confidence and capacity for empathy were at risk during these early years of being a doctor. As your confidence and capacity for empathy plummeted, your risk of burnout, addiction and mental illness began to rise. In desperation, perhaps you worked harder to prove to yourself and everyone else that you belonged; that you were worthy of being a doctor.

For many young doctors this strategy of working harder only serves to prove to themselves how imperfect they are, feeding their internal voice

of doubt and shame, proving to themselves that their primary credential
is 'Imposter'.

Do you recognise these internal voices of imposter, doubt and shame?

> The idea that doctors can suppress their emotions and leave them at
> the door when they come to work is nonsense. Better to learn to use
> them skilfully in the service of everyone's wellbeing.

Medicine has not behaved as if it values its most precious resource,
the doctors providing the care. It has not taught doctors all the skills they
need to do well by their patients, themselves, or each other. Namely the
skills of wellbeing, interpersonal connection and care, and leadership.
Medicine and healthcare more broadly have prioritised the science of
medicine – clinical technical skills – and ignored the art of medicine,
despite the wealth of evidence supporting the need for both in caring,
healing and wellbeing.

## THE HARSH REALITY OF WORKING IN MEDICINE

Occupational Health and Safety laws have not penetrated healthcare like
they have in other industries. Action to ensure occupational health and
safety of doctors as workers has lagged behind many other industries
and has been unbearably slow to change. In recent years many enquiries
have shown:

- high rates of bullying and harassment of junior, female, and
  minority group doctors
- that doctors routinely work long and dangerous hours.

Bullying and harassment are features of the medical landscape.
According to AHPRA's 2020 report, one in three junior doctors reported
having experienced or witnessed harassment or bullying in the previous 12 months. Some hospital departments have lost their training

accreditation due to an inability to meet the expected training guidelines, which has included inappropriate behaviour from some supervising doctors.

Too many doctors continue to work in unsafe conditions in order to advance their career. Working as a junior doctor in a hospital can be harrowing, the exhaustion you have likely experienced is nothing like you could have imagined when you started this journey. Misuse of power is routine in some healthcare workplaces and has prompted several reviews.

Professor of psychology, Dacher Keltner, is the director of the Greater Good Science Centre at the University of California, Berkeley. He has been studying power for decades and has concluded that the costs of powerlessness are profound, amplifying sensitivity to threat, causing hypersensitivity in the stress response and increased cortisol in the body.

> Medicine has many examples where the clear unspoken message about 'the way we do things around here', is a powerful force silencing young doctors and training them to harden up.

If you are a doctor working in a regional or rural area, you may feel unsupported due to a lack of colleagues (workforce shortage). If you have ever called out poor work practices or sought an appeal regarding examination or supervision, you will likely know that these processes are poorly designed and ineffective in many healthcare organisations and need urgent overhaul if doctors are to be well.

> The system and the structure will remain complex and unforgiving. Only you can decide if you are willing to participate and ultimately how you will participate.

As a doctor, you probably expected to work long hours and to meet people who are diseased, disoriented, distressed, depressed, dismembered, disenfranchised and who expect you to help them. You may *not* have expected your employing hospital to ask you to just keep on working indefinitely when there was a workforce gap in the roster. As a primary carer you may not have expected so many dead ends when it came to accessing other services for your patients.

There were significant doctor workforce shortages projected before COVID-19 – there will potentially be more pressure, complexity and unpredictability going forward. COVID-19 has amplified and prioritised the need for healthcare system change. Workforce shortages mean that the way doctors can expect to engage and interact in the future will be different. It will certainly include more teamwork and shared care with other professionals, like nurse practitioners and health coaches. COVID-19 has brought a new urgency in terms of digital health and a confronting reality in terms of workforce shortage, bringing the mental health of doctors and other health professionals into sharp relief.

Whatever effort you have made, you have probably found yourself at some stage during your medical career wondering if it's worth it, and if you'll ever fit in or be good enough for medicine. Finding your place in medicine can be so arduous, planting seeds of doubt about your ability and your belonging, challenging your mental health.

> **Establishing yourself in medicine is a sustained practice in persistence, perseverance, and delayed gratification.**

## THE IMPLICIT MESSAGE OF "DO NO HARM"

The dual systems of healthcare and medicine ask you to put the patient first and to do no harm. While these principals exist for good ethical reason, both principals have implicitly invited you to put yourself second after the patient, both have in part caused harm to doctors.

The obvious example of the relationship between doctor wellbeing and patient safety is the expectation that doctors will work long hours. This causes extreme fatigue and leads to inevitable, predictable errors. You may have done this yourself; stayed at work because there is a patient in front of you, even though you are exhausted. Your fatigue increases your likelihood of error and poor judgement, creating real risk of doing harm to the patient and yourself. Your fatigued brain functions on par with being alcohol effected, giving you limited ability to objectively observe your own behaviour. You are blind to your own unconscious blindness, trained to stay there and keep responding. *Patients first* ringing in your ears.

The system has put everyone in this situation at risk. As the doctor you feel powerless to alter the course of the situation. There is no real way you personally can put the patient first AND ensure you do no harm at the same time. The conditions are clearly not designed for optimal care. Some doctors have passed out mid-procedure due to fatigue and lack of support. In the past, doctors who have tried to call this out have found it to be a career limiting move. The result is everyone has accepted it as the norm, despite the very confronting evidence of increased risk of harm to patients and harm to doctors.

These cultural demands put you in an impossible position. How can you put the patient first and do no harm at the same time, when you have been at work for 14 days in a row with little or no support?

What if we made the foundation principle *safety first* instead?

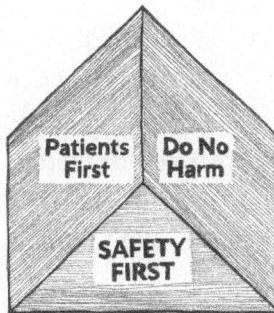

As I write, junior doctors in Australia are launching a class action against their employers for unpaid working hours. These junior doctors are working an average of 16 hours unpaid overtime every week, and half of them say they have made mistakes due to fatigue. This is structural change that unions like the AMA and AMSA have lobbied for over decades. No individual doctor can effect this change across the system, but you can support those in your immediate environment, and you can tell others what's happening to you.

## THE EXTREME TOLL ON YOUR SOUL

It is an irrefutable and distressing fact that working in medicine has led some doctors to take their own lives. The families of these doctors are in no doubt that the work and the working conditions their doctor family member experienced contributed to their death. It doesn't get any more serious than that. These doctors are telling us in the most devastating way that something is not right with the environment they inhabit. Doctor suicide is the worst-case scenario but bears mentioning because of its prevalence across the world, suggesting that there is a systemic problem.

In 2013, a report commissioned by Beyond Blue found that the suicide rate for doctors was higher than any other professional group and higher than the general population rate of suicide in Australia. This was especially so for junior doctors and female doctors. One in ten doctors had had suicidal thoughts in the 12 months prior to the survey. In 2020, researchers at Monash University reviewed more than 60 international studies looking at the prevalence of suicide death, ideation and attempts. They found that some occupations do indeed increase the risk of suicide, and that this is true for female doctors and male nurses.

In the UK, 430 health professionals died from suicide between 2011 and 2015, nearly two people every week. It is estimated 400 doctors die from suicide in the US every year, with junior doctors and female doctors most at risk.

The research also points to doctors experiencing higher rates of depression, anxiety, drug and alcohol misuse and burnout. The Beyond Blue report found that 3.4% of doctors experienced very high levels of psychological distress, much higher than the wider community at 2.6%. Nearly half of young doctors (47.5%) experienced burnout, and female doctors are at much greater risk of mental health issues (depression 27.1%, men 16.6%; anxiety 11.3%, men 6.9%).

> We need an urgent paradigm shift from patient first
> to putting yourself first.

Think of yourself as a passenger on the healthcare system plane. Let the pilot, ground staff and others sort out flying and landing the plane. **For now, make sure you know where your oxygen mask is and how to use it.** You can't help anyone or participate in longer-term systemic change if you are dead or have left the plane altogether. You will contribute much more in the long run if you are alive and well. If it's hard to think of yourself first, try safety first as your guiding principle.

> Put your own oxygen mask on first and understand how to use it,
> without it the situation could be dire.

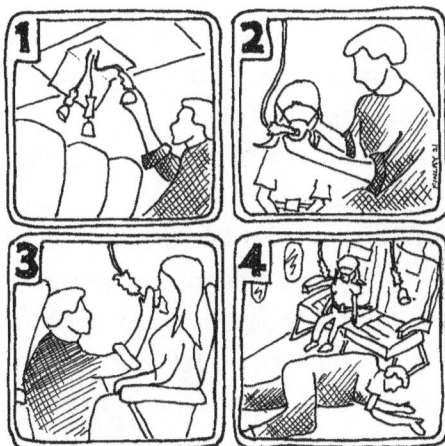

## TAKING CARE OF YOURSELF INTO THE FUTURE

The biggest barriers to seeking help are stigma and fear. The Beyond Blue study found that 59% of responding doctors felt that being a patient would be embarrassing. Doctors who need mental healthcare worry about what their colleagues will think, what their patients will think, and importantly whether such a disclosure will threaten their registration and ongoing ability to practise. Worrying what others will think is innately human. You are human before you are a doctor.

> Relying on the system to change so that you have a better experience of medicine is an entirely unrealistic expectation on your part, one that is disempowered and neglects your own capacity within your own life.

While the systemic issues described in this chapter have a huge impact on the way you practise, they are slow to change. You cannot wait around indefinitely for them to be resolved; your own wellbeing is too important.

There is no shame in leaving medicine if that is the right choice for you – people change jobs and lifestyles all the time. The shame is in the collective missed opportunity to help doctors develop the skills they need to take care of themselves and each other while they do their vital work. Work that the whole community depends on.

Before you throw your hands in the air, blame the system, and make a momentous change in direction, I hope you will see this book as an invitation to pause, take a step back and review what it is you are trying to achieve, why and for whom. Perhaps you can design your medical career differently, so it is more satisfying. Perhaps you can learn the skills you need to achieve a better balance, to relate differently to your environment. Perhaps you can change your relationship to medicine.

> Your capacity, performance, and wellbeing are dependent on the environment you work in and on your personal skills. It is not all about the environment. You can have an influence on your own life.

Let's begin together to focus on you, so that you can learn the extra skills you need to be well for the long term to be a truly effective doctor?

# 2 STOP SURVIVING AND START FLOURISHING

Would you know a thriving doctor if you saw one?

Have you noticed that some of your colleagues seem to suffer more than others in their medical life? Perhaps you've noticed that some of your medical colleagues don't seem to suffer at all because of their work. Some of them even seem to have worked out the work-life balance thing and are enjoying their work.

What are they doing differently?

The World Health Organisation defines health as:

*A state of complete physical, mental and social well-being and not merely the absence of disease or infirmity.*

When the WHO talk about health, they reflect on health as a basic human right that everyone can expect to achieve in the present, and that this state of being in whole self-health creates the best opportunity for ongoing future health.

There is plenty of evidence that the skills of wellbeing can be learnt and that these skills can help you do much more than be well. They can set you up for a long fulfilling career in medicine that is satisfying and even joyful. High performance and wellbeing enable each other. A balanced life can be achieved as you grow your own sense of agency. Once you do the work to build your skills, you will feel empowered to design your best life while you work as a doctor.

## THE SKILLS OF WELLBEING

Martin Seligman was the first psychologist to shift the research frame of psychology from looking at what goes wrong in human mental health and behaviour to asking questions about what goes well. He wanted to know what people with no pathology did that was keeping them well.

Seligman is considered the father of positive psychology, which is an important part of the theoretical basis underpinning coaching. Although he is a self-described pessimist, he has shown that optimism, motivation, and character are important for wellbeing. His published works initially defined positive psychology as being concerned with happiness and satisfaction, and demonstrated by positive emotion, engagement and meaning. As he continued his research, he determined that the key topic of positive psychology is wellbeing, and its goal is to increase human *flourishing*.

> Seligman and others working in positive psychology use the word 'flourishing' to describe positive mental health and overall wellbeing.

Seligman ultimately concluded that there is *no prescription* for wellbeing, rather that positive psychology can *describe* what well people actually do. To describe wellbeing, he settled on the five elements listed below, saying that each element contributes a varying degree to the flourishing of different individuals. Seligman refers to these five measurable elements as **PERMA.**

Take a look at the five elements of PERMA and reflect on how each one plays out for you. Can you think of a time when you felt like you were really flourishing?

How important was each factor in that experience of flourishing?

1. **Positive emotion** – feeling happiness, pleasure, comfort and a sense of life satisfaction.
2. **Engagement** – being in a state of flow as assessed subjectively by you, the experiencer.
3. **Relationships** – feeling connected; we are social animals and do better in each other's company.
4. **Meaning** – belonging to and serving something bigger than yourself.
5. **Accomplishment** – having a sense of achievement and progress in your chosen activity.

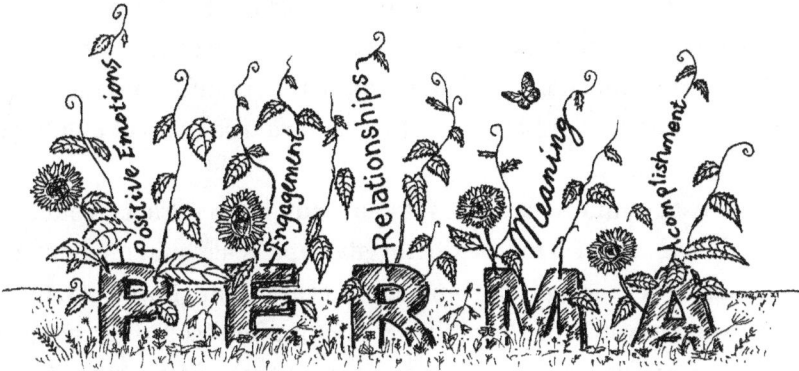

## MOVING TO FLOURISHING

Your state of wellbeing exists on a continuum as shown in the following image (adapted from several other health continuum).

### Wellbeing Continuum

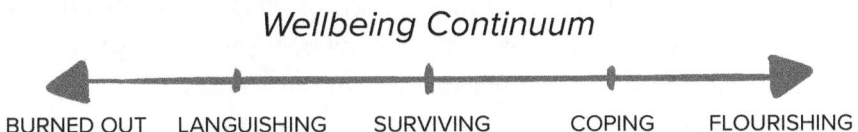

BURNED OUT    LANGUISHING    SURVIVING    COPING    FLOURISHING

Let's consider a little more what each of these states might look like in medical practice:

## 1. Burned out

A burned-out doctor has lost their joy and meaning in work. They feel exhausted, are cynical about most things (especially healthcare), and may also be hostile towards people and things they previously cared deeply about. In this state of being, the doctor feels undervalued, taken for granted, abandoned or ignored, and helpless to do anything about their situation.

A doctor who is burned out has lost their sense of efficacy and, by definition, their sense of agency. They say things like "Who cares?" and "What's the point anyway, it won't make a scrap of difference". Their thinking has become narrow, their emotions are painful, and their capacity to effect change is diminished. This can be a true crisis of identity and meaning for a doctor.

The most common responses to burn out are to retract, avoid and in the worst-case scenario for the doctor, give up. As a result, the doctor will usually take some leave. But burnout is more than simple exhaustion. On returning to work, the burned-out doctor often feels their symptoms again within a very short time, perhaps even with the first patient they see.

## 2. Languishing

Psychologist Corey Keyes defined the opposite of flourishing as *languishing* in 2002, saying this meant an absence of mental health. Keyes described this absence of feeling good about your life as "emptiness and stagnation", experiencing life as "hollow, empty, a shell and a void". Languishing describes a loss of interest in life and is characterised by feeling listless, apathetic and low on energy. Languishing is not a mental illness, but it does describe that feeling of not being as well as you can be, and it does increase your risk of a major depressive episode.

Doctors languishing in their career have told me that they are stuck with little or no career advancement, and little challenge in their life except to remain remotely interested in work that has become dull. Some are frustrated by this. Some have lost all joy or fulfilment in their work and say, "Who cares?".

It is unlikely a doctor who is languishing can motivate others as they are not able to motivate themselves with any consistency. The languishing doctor may feel some sense of their own agency, but they lack the energy to activate it or don't feel connected enough to any sense of purpose to be bothered.

### 3. Surviving

There are lots of metaphors for surviving medicine. The doctor who is surviving looks okay and might even feel okay some of the time, but they are like a duck paddling frantically under the water. When someone describes themselves as surviving, they are actively engaged in their work and generally have lots of energy. However, this person is acutely aware that they are spending more energy than they are creating. This leaves them depleted and they may not be fully functioning as a result. They feel in need of time or space for rest and recovery but feel thwarted by the demands placed upon them.

In survival mode, doctors are more aware of their risk of making a mistake and will comment on their fatigue, their sense of imminent collapse and question how much longer they can keep working like this. This mode of operating has been lauded in medicine, worn like a badge of honour. Surviving medicine is seen as an achievement, but it is not sustainable. These doctors feel frustrated that they do not have their work-life balance worked out and guilty that they should be able to do more. For some it's more work and for others it's more activity or time away from work. These doctors likely experience some of the PERMA elements in their life sometimes.

### 4. Coping

People who are coping are engaged in their own life. These people are actively seeking ways to manage themselves within their context. These doctors are able to invest in themselves, to consciously choose how they think, feel and behave. They believe in principle that they can meet the demands of their life or find the resources they need to be able to do so.

Coping skills help you deal with the stress in your life. When you are able to do this, you usually feel better psychologically and physically.

A coping state implies you are managing the realities of your life for the most part. A doctor who is coping will be more likely engaged in their work, giving it their energy *and* also feeling energised by it. A coping mindset is one of personal agency. The doctor is able to feel their own influence and impact some of the time in their work and their life. The five elements of PERMA are probably experienced by the doctor who is coping at least some of the time.

Some coping behaviours are better than others, so it is important to enquire about *how* you are coping. Strategies that give quick relief but do not really attend to the problem might be considered more survival strategies than coping strategies. For example, misuse of alcohol and drugs is a poor coping strategy; asking for help is an example of a useful coping strategy.

## 5. Flourishing

Felicia Huppert and Timothy So from the University of Cambridge defined flourishing as "the experience of life going well" with a "combination of feeling good and functioning effectively". A flourishing person has high emotional, psychological, and social wellbeing. The simplest way for you to establish if you are flourishing is to ask yourself- what makes me truly happy? And then reflect on how much of the time you feel this way. Other words that might help you describe your personal experience of flourishing include thriving, prospering, growing well, and blossoming.

A person who is flourishing is fully engaged in their own life, empowered to create a life that makes them feel subjectively happy much of the time. Their life is a demonstration of the five PERMA elements in action – positive emotions, engagment, clear meaning, achievement and positive relationships. This does not mean there is no challenge, discomfort or adversity in their life. It means that the flourishing person is well resourced internally and has the support network to allow them to respond effectively to whatever life throws at them.

The flourishing adult has a variety of interests and the energy to pursue them. They are responsible and accountable for their life, including their self-care, and they are aware of their internal and external environments, responding to them constructively.

A flourishing doctor is upbeat, enjoys their work, feels like they have got the work-life balance sorted more often than not, is committed to partnering and collaborating with others, values their relationships, is emotionally in tune, and has a 'can do' mindset most of the time. They are able to manage their own internal responses to their work as well as the external environment (including the complexities of healthcare) effectively. These doctors are empowered and fulfilled. They can feel their own agency in their life, and they use it to create more wellbeing for themselves and those around them. **They are thriving**.

It is important to clarify that flourishing is not the opposite of mental illness. A person can have a diagnosis of a mental illness and still flourish.

> **When you are flourishing, you have more discretionary effort to give, you connect with others more easily and you feel more empowered and fulfilled. Your medical career is more sustainable when you are flourishing.**

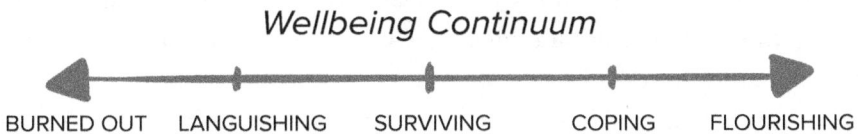

## Wellbeing Continuum

BURNED OUT    LANGUISHING    SURVIVING    COPING    FLOURISHING

## Reflection

You can make a rudimentary assessment now. Take a pen and make three marks as follows on the Wellbeing Continuum:

1.    Where would you place yourself on this wellbeing continuum today?
2.    Where would you like to be?
3.    Where would you put showing up but not really being present or engaged (being on autopilot)?

None of the points on this continuum show mental illness, all are descriptions of how you feel subjectively in your mind and body about your life. Your wellbeing is dynamic and can change over time depending on what is happening in your life.

- What do you notice about your three marks on the continuum?
- How often are you living near mark number 3 - near to your autopilot mark?
- How often are you living near mark number 2 - where you would like to be?
- What action are you willing to take to live more often near mark number 2?

Some people describe medicine as a grind culture. When you are barely surviving, that's all you can do – show up each day and hope you can survive another shift grinding out another day on autopilot. You probably know some people who have burned out and some who have left medicine altogether. This is an indictment on the system we have for training doctors and on medicine itself. The estimated cost of training and onboarding a doctor in Australia in 2017 was $451,000. Estimates for consultants in the US vary from US$450,000 - $1.1m. What a waste to see any individual or community make that sort of investment and not reap the rewards when there are measures we could take to make a doctor's life so much better.

If this is you, make the decision now to get the help you need to be well. Forget about what is best for medicine, your patients, your colleagues, or your organisation. Turn your full attention to your own wellbeing, invest in yourself, and everyone will ultimately benefit. No one is benefiting while you grind out the days languishing and burning out.

Your place on the Wellbeing Continuum is subject to change. Your wellbeing is dynamic. If there is a gap between where you have assessed your wellbeing to be today and where you would really like it to be, know that even small changes in the way you think and behave can help you move along the continuum in a short time.

> Most doctors have room for improvement when it comes to
> wellbeing – how about you?

## WHAT BEHAVIOURS WILL CULTIVATE WELLBEING?

Richard Davidson, founder and director of the Centre for Healthy Minds at the University of Wisconsin-Madison, is a neuroscientist who has also investigated this central question of why some people are well. The Dalai Lama asked him in 1992 why scientists couldn't harness the tools of modern neurobiology to study virtuous qualities such as kindness and compassion.

Davidson and his team did exactly that. Since then, they have concluded that:

> Wellbeing is a skill that can be developed.

At the 2016 Wisdom 2.0 conference held at UCLA Berkeley, Davidson described four constituents of wellbeing that his team had neuro-scientifically validated. They have been able to identify the neurological circuits of these four constituents and measure how they change over time in relation to an individual's actions.

They have found that these circuits exhibit neuroplasticity, meaning that they can be shaped through training and experience. You can intentionally take responsibility for your brain developing your wellbeing by what you choose to practise, instead of unwittingly practising habits (behaviours and thinking patterns) that do not support your wellbeing.

Here are the four constituent behaviours defined by Davidson and his team that they suggest you cultivate for your own wellbeing.

1.  Resilience – the rapidity with which you recover from adversity. People who have more rapid recovery from adversity, who get back to baseline quicker, have more wellbeing. You can modulate this circuitry with regular formal mindfulness practice. The

research so far suggests you will need a lot of practice to make this change visible in your brain circuitry, but nevertheless it can be done. The key here is regular practice, 10 minutes every day is a useful goal. Regularly activating the neuronal connections makes them more efficient.

2.  Outlook – having a positive outlook for the world, being able to recognise the innate basic goodness in others and being able to savour positive experiences. People with depression show activation in this circuitry but it is fleeting. People with more wellbeing have more extended circuit activation. Loving kindness meditation (metta) can alter this circuitry quite quickly with a relatively modest dose of practice. Davidson's team have seen this circuitry change in randomised trial research within two weeks at 30 mins of practice per day. These circuitry changes were also predictive of pro-social behaviour, helping people connect.

3.  Attention – maintaining your attention on the activity you are currently doing. Killingsworth and Gilbert have demonstrated that a wandering mind is an unhappy mind, with adults not paying attention to what they're doing 47% of the time they are awake. Davidson and many others have demonstrated that contemplative practices like mindful meditation are vehicles for changing the neurocircuits for attention so that focus improves.

4.  Generosity – engaging in generous and altruistic behaviours activates circuits in the brain that are key to fostering wellbeing and are more enduring than other kinds of positive incentives. In other words, kindness towards others activates wellbeing circuits.

Neuroplasticity is going on all the time whether you notice or not. Be intentional; you have more control over your wellbeing than you know. To be intentional takes effort and energy. Davidson invites us all to turn the same amount of attention to intentionally developing our brains as we do to brushing our teeth. The data shows a few minutes a day makes a difference, changing your brain circuitry to be more able to help you to be well.

His research has found that these practices in mindfulness, savouring, and generosity have an impact on people's epigenetics, systemic biology, and physical health. In his most recent talks, he has pointed to awareness, connection, insight and purpose as the way to cultivate wellbeing.

Your positive and negative experiences and emotions all contribute to your understanding of the world, in fact the best things in life almost always include positive *and* negative emotions. Childbirth is a classic example. Avoiding adversity and challenge and seeking perfectionism is not the route to wellbeing or high performance. It's more effective to approach life with optimism, hope, strong relationships and purpose.

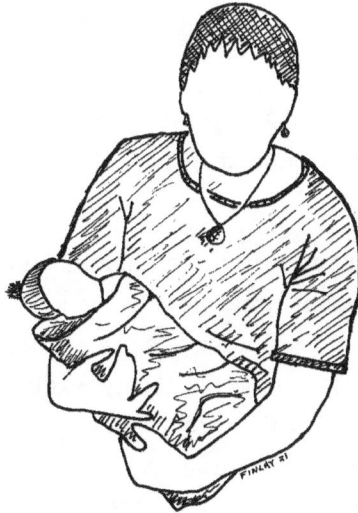

Experiencing adversity in your training and work in medicine creates many opportunities to learn and grow. Getting comfortable with being on your learning edge is an important capacity, I often tell the doctors I work with to *get comfortable with being uncomfortable*. This also applies to the emotions you are feeling. However, this does not ever apply to being bullied, harassed or humiliated in any way. Before we get to how you build your skills, it's important to consider psychological safety and to discuss power.

## PSYCHOLOGICAL SAFETY

> Competition, perfectionism, cultural requirements to never show emotion or ask for help, and deep hierarchy all serve to maintain clear power differentials in medicine.

Across medicine, power grows as you progress up the hierarchy, though this has not necessarily been true for certain marginalised or minority groups. If you are further up the hierarchical ladder, it is incumbent on you to create systems and structures that improve the psychological safety of those you work with.

Even the most skilled and empowered junior doctor can only make a small difference to the psychological safety of their organisation because they are:

- highly mobile working on rotation and short-term contracts, seeking the next job or placement
- dependent on their supervisor's grace, good will, teaching, time and attention to learn technical skills and to endorse their competencies for further progression
- often overwhelmed by the steep learning curve they are on, constantly being asked to prove their capacity as they move through the various hurdles to advance their careers without adding extra obligations to their daily work.

Every member of a healthcare team can and should make a positive difference to psychological safety in the workplace. However, if you are disempowered and busy keeping yourself safe, be patient and commit to making this positive difference in the future when you have the skills and the capacity. For now, do whatever you need to do to keep yourself safe and please do these three things:

1.  Start building and strengthening your support network around you, connecting with people you trust wherever they are, sharing with them some of what you are experiencing.
2.  If you are being bullied or harassed this is NEVER okay. Tell people what is happening, contact the appropriate work-related support agents and discuss your options – you'll find a list of support resources on our website: www.coachingfordoctors.net.au
3.  Start practising self-compassion, especially in your self-talk.

> **Psychological safety is essential for people to truly flourish.**

According to Tim Clark, author of '*The 4 Stages of Psychological Safety*,' we are better able to flourish when we are participating in a cooperative system. Although healthcare is a team sport in its delivery to patients, it is a competitive environment for most doctors every day. Not just in training, also in private practice, in terms of status and prestige which effects referral, access to resources like theatre lists, promotion and professional esteem. This is also true for the many doctors engaged in research who are competing for resources, funding, and esteem.

Clark describes the four stages of psychological safety that build on each other as follows:

1.  Inclusion Safety – allowed into the club, as it were, a genuine invitation to participate. Inclusion safety is a matter of life and death for humans, we have a deep psychological need to belong. Young doctors are continually checking themselves to make sure they are behaving in the ways that will keep them accepted by other doctors. Medicine has created many training mechanisms and other opportunities for junior doctors to feel vulnerable about whether they will continue to be accepted by the medicine club. The social norms are powerful and unforgiving. If the doctor is not able to compete, harden up and strive for perfectionism, they are unlikely to feel good enough. This

threatens their sense of belonging and being accepted and has had dire consequences for thousands of doctors, many of whom have tragically taken their own lives.

2.  Learner Safety – facilitates learning, including asking questions and for help without fear of retribution. Mistakes are welcome and expected as part of the learning process. "Safe passage to learning opens [sic] the buds of potential, cultivating confidence, resilience and independence", Clark says. In this environment, learners can stretch themselves, test their capacity and self-efficacy, start feeling their own autonomy.

    A young doctor working in this environment has more opportunity to flourish and be well, feeling empowered and experiencing their own agency. This is the environment to cultivate and foster in healthcare so that doctors can flourish as they learn.

3.  Contributor Safety – offers open access to fully participate in the environment with autonomy. The doctor's contribution is still dependent on the leader and the team's encouragement. To date, I have met very few doctors who have described working in such an environment.

4.  Challenger Safety – welcoming challenges to the status quo without any reprisal or personal risk. Doctors who work in such a safe environment will likely feel confident in themselves and in all of those around them. This is the kind of space that allows true creativity, which is precious and rare in healthcare. Medicine will need a huge transformation for these workplaces to exist.

It is likely that you are working in level one conditions in Clark's framework of psychological safety, meaning that you have been accepted into the club and are allowed to participate in medicine, so long as you comply with the established norms of behaviour:

- Compete fiercely, work harder than anyone around you if possible.

- Always strive for perfection.
- Demonstrate a toughness that is called 'resilience' but really means 'never show weakness, never ask for help, and don't expect help because no one has the capacity to give you any'.
- Show as little emotion as possible, preferably none.
- Accept the status quo.

**A note on power, influence, and imposter syndrome.**

Jeffrey Pfeffer is Professor of Organizational Behaviour at the Graduate School of Business at Stanford University. He has spent his life studying power and influence. He says in his book '*Power*', "Belief that the world is a *just* place anaesthetises people to the need to be proactive in building a power base". This, as a result, limits their ability to influence.

He encourages every adult to seek power as if their life depended on it. This goes to the heart of personal agency. It is important that you understand your own power, both for your *self* and in your *role* as a doctor seeking to collaborate with patients and colleagues. We will look at self and role in more detail in chapter 4.

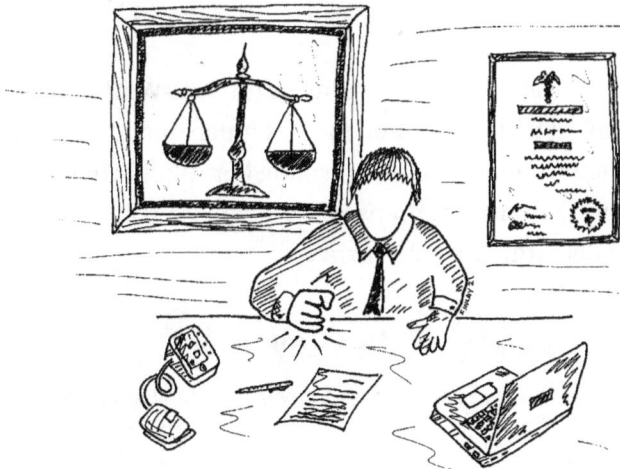

The Just-World Hypothesis was first described by Melvin Lerner, who said that people wanted to think the world was predictable and comprehensible and therefore potentially controllable.

> The Just-World Hypothesis shows that collectively we believe that people, by and large, get what they deserve.

Good people will be rewarded, bad people will be punished. If a person has prospered, they are considered to have been good and to have caused their prosperity. Just-world thinking also holds the reverse to be true; that when something awful happens, the person must have done something to have caused it.

Are you applying this kind of thinking to your own life? If you are burdened with imposter syndrome, you are caught in beliefs that you *should* be something more than what you are, that you are unworthy, not good enough or even that you are somehow bad and deserving of your problems. If you truly believe this narrative, it may be the root of your lack of agency.

Sometimes things go badly for reasons beyond you.

> You are not in control of everything. You have a choice about how you respond, about how you think, and even about how you feel.

Imposter syndrome finds its origins in the Just-World Hypothesis. It ignores the element of luck and that there is much outside an individual's control. As a doctor, you may be aware of the Just-World Hypothesis when you think of your patients, perhaps you are able to recognise that MND (ALS) does not discriminate for instance.

## Reflection

- Do you have the same awareness for how you think about your own life?
- Do you recognise and remember that no matter how hard you work, who you network with and how many high distinctions and awards you receive, a great many things are still outside of your control?
- Do you attribute any of your success to luck?

- Do you remember to pay homage and feel grateful for all those who have helped you in your career and in your life?
- Do you think of your whole life as one big collaboration? Or do you beat yourself up for not being good enough?
- Do you let your inner critic run rampant?

> **Recognise that it is not a just or fair world. You have the capacity to design your life within a context, you do not have the capacity to control all the variables in your world.**

You do have the capacity to choose how you respond, to be account-able for those choices and to take responsibility for yourself. Thank you for taking the time to learn and to build the skills you need to do well and be well as you work in the uncertain, difficult, risky world of medicine.

Amy Edmonson PhD is the Professor of Leadership and Management at Harvard Business School and she also happens to be married to a physician. She is one of the world's leading researchers and practitioners in psychological safety. She says that impression manage-ment at work is second nature. Humans use it for self protection from a young age, and it often limits our learning; it can impact negatively on patient safety.

Edmonson defines psychological safety as a belief that this workplace is safe for speaking up and when I do it will be valued by my colleagues. In other words there is permission for candor. She continues saying that psychological safety is not about being nice, touchy-feely, a licence to whine or a guarantee that all your ideas will be applauded; it's not a trigger-free space. Rather it is an obligation to dissent in engaging, pro-ductive ways in the service of the goal of excellence in a volatile, complex and uncertain world.

If you lead others in healthcare it is your duty to learn about how you can create increasing psychological safety in your workplace. If you are a doctor training others or leading teams you need to know that people working in psychologically safe teams manage risk more effectively and are safer for workers and patients. I hope you can keep these ideas in mind as you read on. Leadership that builds psychologically safe teams values humility, curiosity, empathy and is willing to help. It's not so much what you do, but how you do it. As a doctor you are inevitably in the role of leader sometimes.

# 3 | REGULATE YOURSELF

Clara's
Story

*Clara came to Australia in her early twenties. She owned her GP practice with her husband, and a further 15 associates worked there. Her children were at university and life was full. Despite all this, Clara found herself feeling burned out. At the point she came to me for coaching, she had been a practising GP for 25 years.*

*Although she loved her patients, many of whom she had known for a long time, she was fed up with the rudeness she often experienced. They expected her to do whatever they asked and had no regard for her clinical judgement. On top of that, she was weighed down by a host of other factors, such as being tired, the burden of the administrative needs of her business, being fed up with people asking her where she was from, and the current lack of collegiality between the doctors in her practice. This was making her feel less tolerant of these entitled patients than she normally would be.*

*One of the first things I asked her to do was to start noticing and naming her thoughts and feelings. She noticed her mood was low and her emotions were erratic, especially with her practice manager and at home. Clara also described her inner critic as too noisy. We discussed starting a mindfulness habit to build her ability to manage all these challenging inputs. Clara was curious about mindfulness, saying that she had read lots of books about it, but didn't really understand how it applied to her or how it could help her at work.*

*We started working together, discussing how she could intersperse mindful moments throughout her day, using her feet, her breath, and her patients as her anchors. In addition, she started using a meditation app for five minutes daily, and she met with a meditation teacher to practise and talk about her experience with meditation. This committed action, experimenting, and practising over a few weeks allowed Clara to test and reflect. Learning in the supportive environment of coaching helped her remain accountable to her own goals.*

*Three years on, she describes herself as focused and steady and she enjoys her work. Clara credits her mindfulness practice and the time she committed to coaching with helping her fall in love with medicine again. She feels reconnected with her own intention, and able to weather the challenges of a busy and vibrant GP practice.*

## WHAT DOES SELF-REGULATION MEAN?

> **Self-regulation is the ongoing ability to maintain your physical, psychological and emotional balance.**

As a doctor, you work in a complex, fast paced, changing environment. You regularly interact with hundreds of people in a single day, there are lots of factors you are not in control of and an enormous amount of information to remember and process. Thankfully, your body automatically and continuously takes care of most things without any conscious direction from you. Your heart and lungs keep working and your mind keeps generating hypotheses and making associations, all keeping you safe and alive.

Your capacity to achieve at work is dependent on your ability to:

- maintain your focus and clarity
- balance achieving tasks and maintaining relationships
- meet the needs of others while remaining aware of your own needs when you are under pressure.

Your ongoing self-regulation in the face of ever-changing circumstances is the foundation of your wellbeing and your performance in the immediate and the longer term.

> **The opposite of self-regulation is dysregulation; feeling overwhelmed, confused, undermined, unaware, out of balance and out of control.**

To be a great doctor and a well person, you need to be able to regulate your complex internal environment – your *self*. Your mind is what you use to regulate your self. When I use that word – mind – I include all of your body, not just your brain.

To improve your self-regulation skills, you must do your own push ups. No one else can do them for you and reading a book won't get you there either. Self-regulation is an inside job which requires skill and practice, a little bit often is the best way. As these practices become routine habits, your internal scaffold strengthens, creating a foundation from which you can thrive. Often, the work of the coach is to help keep you accountable as you embed these practices.

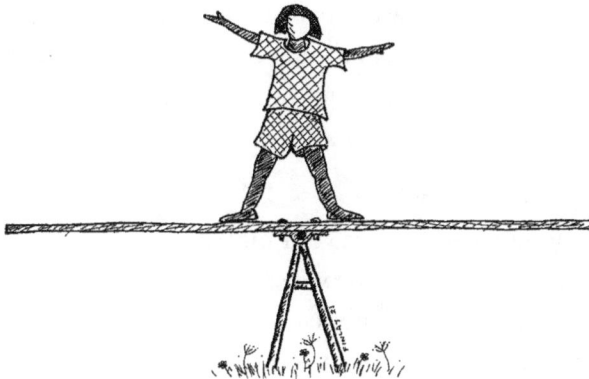

Picture an old-fashioned seesaw, not the modern kind with the big springs underneath, but the kind that would crash to the ground if your playmate suddenly jumped off!

I remember learning to balance one of those seesaws as a child by standing in the middle in exactly the right place. Shifting my weight in minute movements until both ends were just right, balanced. The second I lost focus, I was either falling off or adapting and adjusting my body in tiny ways to meet the conditions.

> Balancing your complex life as a doctor requires your ongoing attention and awareness.

Holding your balance in the constantly changing environment of healthcare requires your constant adjusting and adapting to manage the risk of falling. The key is in *noticing* that the conditions have changed, inside your body or outside your body, so that you can make the appropriate adjustments in time.

> The more you work with your internal locus of control, the more capacity you will have for success, the more empowered you will feel.

Regulating yourself begins with what you notice in your internal environment, what you are aware of. As you tune in and become more intentionally curious, you change what you notice, giving you more options.

Pause for a moment now to notice what you are aware of in this moment:

- your physical body
- your thoughts and where your mental attention is
- your emotions and all the sensations, physiology and the thinking that accompanies them
- your values, what matters to you
- your beliefs and how they create biases in you
- remembering that there are things you don't control and lots of things outside of your awareness that affect you too.

What you pay attention to and what you are aware of determines your experience of the world. The good news is that you can alter what you pay attention to and are aware of. But you need to tune in and *notice* what you are doing. Only then can you make changes for your benefit and ultimately the benefit of your patients.

As you build your attention and awareness skills, you can fortify and finesse your internal environment so that you have a stronger base to take better care of yourself. Bit by bit, you will change your experience in ways that empower you to be a better doctor and to live your best life. Your mind is directing your internal environment, creating your reality. For example, becoming aware of the impact of your negative self-talk allows you to do something about it, to learn the skills to change your mindset.

> **When you can regulate yourself, you can maintain your balance and free up your energy to create the kind of career and life you want. Use your personal agency where it counts.**

## THREE SKILL SETS FOR SELF-REGULATION

Beyond sleep, nutrition, and movement, there are three core skill-sets that are interrelated, listed below. You can develop these to regulate your self.

1. Clarity of mind
2. Emotional literacy
3. Self-awareness

> **Only when you are aware of your thoughts, emotions, and behaviours can you start to examine, test and change them.**

These self-regulation skills don't develop accidentally. Like all skill development, intentional practice is key. Let's explore each of these skill sets in more detail so you can start practising and improving your self-regulation.

## 1. CLARITY OF MIND

Clarity of mind is predominantly about mindfulness, however there's a foundational regulatory process that we need to make sure we're getting right first. And that's sleep.

### Sleep

Sleep affects your wellbeing and your performance positively. Along with nutrition and movement, it is a pillar for good health.

The American National Sleep Foundation and Australia's Sleep Health Foundation concur that adults need 7-9 hours of sleep per night for optimum health, wellbeing, safety and performance. As a doctor, you may need to be flexible about your sleep. Depending on your roster, on call duties and speciality, you may need to include naps in your routine which are well supported in the research. Your sleep routine will be specific to you, the important thing to notice is that for you to develop good internal regulation, attention and awareness skills, you need an adequate amount of good quality sleep. When you don't have it, your body has to work much harder to keep you regulated.

About half of the adult population is sleep deprived. Most doctors have some on-call responsibilities undermining their opportunity for optimal sleep. The effects of sleep deprivation can be seen after just a day or two. After 48 hours of being awake, you will feel very fatigued, your brain will start going into brief periods of unconsciousness (0.5 – 15 second periods known as microsleep). Three or four days without sleep will cause you to start hallucinating.

Without enough sleep, you are likely to be more irritable, less fun to be around, your judgement is likely to be cloudier, your reaction time slower, and your ability to make decisions impaired. With enough sleep deprivation, you will become dysregulated.

Lack of sleep is an amplifying stressor, making all the other stressors seem worse. It reduces your energy levels and your prosocial positive feelings, interferes with your ability to remain self-aware, pay attention, have clarity of mind, and regulate your internal systems, including your emotions. Lack of sleep impacts your mood, making you more vulnerable to stress and burnout.

Disturbed sleep can be a bit of a chicken and egg dilemma. Sometimes it's about resolving sleep habits and hygiene, other times it's about resolving another problem that then allows you to relax and go to sleep. Sleep helps you modulate the impact of stressors in your life, which in turn helps you sleep.

As a doctor, you rely on your decision-making skills, your role as a problem solver, and your energy. Poor sleep or lack of sleep diminishes your capacities, reducing your performance and limiting your effectiveness. As your effectiveness, capacity and wellbeing declines, you will find it more and more difficult to encourage and support your patients, colleagues, and yourself. Everything gets harder, including maintaining your hopeful, empowered and energetic mindset and attitude.

> **It's more difficult to strengthen your attention and awareness skills if you don't get enough quality sleep.**

Practising mindfulness has also been shown to improve sleep, just as sleep improves our ability to be mindful.

## Mindfulness

So many doctors have started this work to train their attention and grow their self-awareness saying, "I don't really do mindfulness, I don't see how it can make a difference". They have misunderstood the impact of training their attention and raising their awareness.

> **Mindfulness helps you notice things you had no awareness of before, creating more choice for you. Feeling like you have a choice reduces your stress, increases your sense of empowerment and agency, and helps you achieve balance.**

Clarity of mind is achieved by being aware of where your attention is and then managing that attention. Managing your attention looks like this:

Choose what to focus on, pay attention to it.

1.  Notice (awareness) that you are distracted from the chosen focus.
2.  Bring your attention back to the chosen focus.
3.  Maintain attention by repeating over and over again.

This clarity of mind means that you remain aware of the other possibilities inside you and around you, but you remain focused on the task at hand. As you train your mind you are distracted less, and you can maintain your focus for longer.

> The most powerful way to build your clarity of mind is
> by practising mindfulness.

Mindfulness means bringing your full attention to the present moment on purpose without judgement. When you are mindful, you are fully engaged in one thing; you have awareness of the environment around you but you are not distracted by it. You are attentive *and* aware.

In mindfulness, you use your energy to notice what is, not to judge what ought to be, should be, or might be. Mindfulness is neither optimistic nor pessimistic, it is being present to what is. This non-judgemental quality of mindfulness opens the space for you to learn, to gain insight, and to become aware.

As you learn about yourself and raise your awareness, you tune in, carefully adjusting, purposefully listening, and finding just the right movement. Like balancing a seesaw, you need to notice where your energy is going in real time, in any given context, and be able to adjust.

To create work-life balance, you need to know what you are *already* doing and what it is you'd like to be doing: this is the core of personal agency and self-awareness. To find out, you need to sometimes stop *doing* and practise *being*. It is in being that we can notice. No change occurs without noticing.

---

## ACTIVITY 1

### Envisage your best life and start noticing what you are doing

Building new habits of regulation is effortful. It is hard to sustain the work of habit change to better regulate yourself if you don't know why you would bother or what you are aiming for in the first place. Learning to practise mindfulness can sometimes make things feel worse before they get better because all the things you were ignoring or denying are now in sharp focus.

Many doctors have been able to tell me easily what they don't want in their lives: I don't have a very kind on-call roster, I don't want to work in the private sector, I don't want to work with heartsink patients, I can't reduce my hours because there is no one else to see the patients. They find it harder to tell me what they do want in their lives or their work.

To achieve balance in your life, start imagining what a great week *could* or *would* look like. Don't limit yourself with the current boundaries of time or money. Take out a sheet of paper and write a list of all the activities you would *like* to do regularly: daily or weekly. Use the guide below. Now write another list of the activities you would like to do occasionally. Now prioritise the two lists into 'essential' and 'nice to have'. Take a few minutes to sit contemplating your lists. We can look at this again in the next chapter. For now, experience whatever arises in your body, notice any resistance you have in your thinking, any tension in your body and write down what you notice in the third box.

Every reaction is valid and welcome, there is no right or wrong answer, **you are simply noticing yourself and your life** for a few minutes. As you read this book and other things come into your awareness, come back and add them to your best-life word picture.

**What would you like your best-life balance to include?**

| Regular - Weekly | Occasional - Monthly/ quarterly/ yearly |
|---|---|
| Essential | Essential |
| Nice to Have | Nice to Have |
| Reactions to this exercise | Reactions to this exercise |

Another way to think about this is to ask yourself what brings the most meaning to your life? If this question causes more activities to come into your awareness, add them to the appropriate list.

In the exercise, I asked you to name what you would *like* in your life and then to notice your *reaction* to these preferences and wishes. I'm inviting you to notice what is here in your mind and body right now. If you couldn't name anything that's okay, there are a lot of skills you can develop to improve your capacity and your balance in the chapters ahead. Most of us have plenty of room to improve these skills. **The work of high performance and sustained wellbeing begins with noticing.** Tune in with curiosity, courage, and self-compassion.

> **Noticing is amplified when we are still, when we pause, when we choose to be with what is here, in reality, in this moment.**

It is in being *willing* to choose to *be with* what's actually here that you have the opportunity to notice what is going on. The mindful qualities of acceptance, curiosity, patience, presence and non-judgement create the right environment to learn what is happening in your mind and body, to learn what you need and to notice what you value most.

Viktor Frankl, Austrian neurologist, psychiatrist and holocaust survivor, said, "Between every stimulus and response there is a space. In that space is our power to choose our response. In our response lies our growth and our freedom". Frankl credits this insight with helping him manage the environment of Auschwitz. You can also use it to help you manage the environment of healthcare.

> **Your response to the stimulus makes all the difference.**

Neurologically speaking, if you are not paying attention mindfully with awareness, you are operating in your default network. This is the brain network of habit. Habituated behaviours are fantastic in many ways because they are energy conserving. Researchers estimate that about 40% of our daily behaviours are habituated. It can take anywhere from 18 to 254 days to establish a habit.

This means that walking and talking, driving a car, and many of your well-practised behaviours are cognitively efficient, they do not need much of your energy. It also means that you have tuned out from much of your daily experience. When people are under pressure from hunger, anger, loneliness, lateness, tiredness, stress, or sickness (HALLTSS), they are more likely to revert to default patterns of behaviour – habits – as a means of conserving energy.

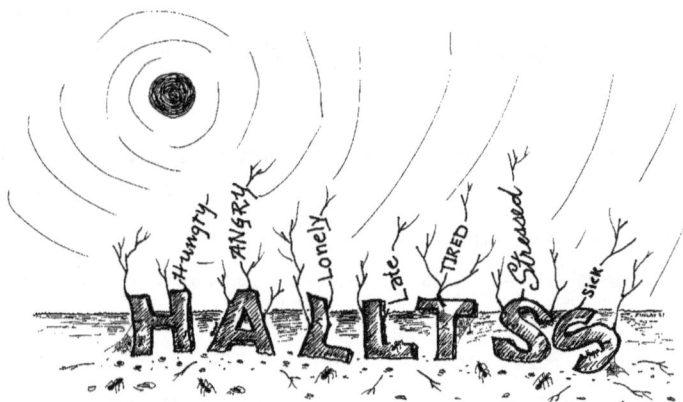

While habits are useful and energy-saving, this 'autopilot' mode can also result in you being distant and disengaged from patients, colleagues and even your own goals and values. Routine and habit help us do many procedural actions well, but they can also create blind spots. If you are depleted by HALLTSS, your body is already working hard to keep you regulated. In this state you are not going to show up as your best doctor. In this state you are more likely to choose the quick and easy route rather than delay your gratification in the service of a longer-term goal. You are more susceptible to cognitive traps like confirmation bias, availability bias, and diagnosis momentum.

Hundreds of doctors have described working while they experienced HALLTSS to me. They have described having little awareness of what was happening at the time and have only seen their poorer decision making in the context of their depleted state in hindsight. Even though they acknowledge that it's not good for them or their patients, this social norm of continuing to work is powerful. Several ED consultants have told me that even on a 12 hour shift they cannot leave the floor for anything - including the toilet or for food or drink - if it is busy. Naming these habits in coaching has led these doctors to change their habits in ways that have improved *their* experience of working as an emergency doctor and team leader. And these doctors have told me later that they believe their patients have a better healthcare experience as a result. They are more regulated and are therefore better doctors, better colleagues, and better people (in their own words).

When you practise mindfulness, you are not putting on your rosy glasses, you are not practising forced positivity, you are facing the reality of what is here right now. In mindfulness you turn towards your experiences, accepting whatever is here in each moment. You are choosing to be aware and pay attention to *all* your experiences, improving your self-awareness, creativity, and choice. You are recognising choice and being accountable for it.

You don't have to like all of your experiences. Avoidance is a valid choice, but you do it with awareness. You can think of your mind as either approaching or avoiding each moment. You either stay with and lean into an experience, or you step back. Both strategies are valuable and can help us survive and thrive if we use them to their best advantage.

Mindfulness is an approach process helping us stay with what is important even when it might be uncomfortable. To use approach and avoid strategies effectively, we need to notice which one we are using and be aware of what is going on in our internal environment.

> **As a problem solver, this clarity of mind has significant benefits to you in your doctor role.**

You are probably very skilled at paying attention and maintaining your awareness in an emergency. If the person in front of you has just stopped breathing, you are probably able to give them your absolute full attention and in that moment you are probably acutely aware of the potential consequences for you and the non-breather. You are possibly also very aware of who else is present, what the noises are around you, perhaps even your own heartbeat or breath. Say you resuscitate the person successfully – fantastic, thank you.

What happens next to your attention and your awareness?

## Reflection

- Do you stay tuned in to your heartbeat or your breath?
- How long does that attention and awareness of your own physiology last?
- Do you move on to the next activity and quickly forget about what happened, ignoring any residual physiological effects?
- Do you start thinking about all the other resuscitations you've been involved in?
- Does this event trigger a memory or does your mind run away with a new story birthed out of this event?
- Where is your attention and your awareness after the event and are you able to redirect your attention and awareness as you wish?
- Do you think about it later in the day?
- What specifically stays with you and what do you do with it?
- Are you able to focus your attention, bring clarity of mind and remain aware when it is not a life and death situation?

> You are most effective in your life when you are fully present to your experience in the moment, noticing, being with whatever is present.
> **All of it.**

In emergencies in your role as doctor, you have been paying attention, acutely aware. You have the skills. Do you want to apply them across all parts of your life?

Mindfulness is an empowering practice that allows you to choose how you respond skilfully. You cannot take any skilful action until you are aware of what is happening. A person who misuses alcohol does not change their behaviour until after they notice and name it as a problem. You did not improve your medical skills by saying '*Yes, I can do everything already*'.

Can you remember when you first started looking inside ears and trying to decide if there was an ear infection or not? Could you diagnose all ear infections in people of all skin colours instantly? Unlikely. More likely you had to practise looking inside lots of different ears, you probably asked for guidance, you possibly asked someone else to look inside some of those ears to decipher and diagnose. You gradually named what you needed to know and do, progressively finessing your skills, refining what you were looking for, asking different questions. As you noticed and named what you needed, you gave yourself the opportunity to improve.

Mindfulness allows you to choose actions that serve your purpose, your intention. You are not in control of every stimulus in your internal or external environment. You can be in control of your response if you learn how to notice and name what is happening at any given moment. Are you willing to apply the same learning attitude and process you used to learn to diagnose ear infections as a junior doctor to learning about yourself?

> **As you build the habit of skilfully noticing what is happening moment-to-moment, you strengthen your capacity to regulate yourself. If you are better able to regulate yourself, you have more energy for making your intentions become reality.**

Learning the skills of mindfulness will allow you to respond more flexibly to your experiences and free up some of your energy. People who have a regular mindfulness practice report feeling less stressed, experience improved relationships and more satisfaction in their work. Physiologically, their immune systems function better, their variable heart rate is improved, and their blood pressure is lower.

Mindfulness, with its qualities of curiosity, non-judgement and kindness, facilitates compassion. Self-compassion helps you to regulate your internal dialogue, softening your self-talk and helping you respond more effectively to the external environment. Your relationship with yourself, others, and *the system* is transformed. Compartmentalising has yet to be shown to offer all of these benefits, to my knowledge.

Keep compartmentalising and suppression as ONE of your self-regulation skills. My invitation to you is to be curious about what else you can add to your skillset so that you can be as effective as you can be, so that your performance and wellbeing potential is raised rather than limited.

### How to train clarity of mind

You can apply mindful practice to practically every activity you participate in, it doesn't have to be an added extra to an already busy day. You can start building your attention muscle with any activity. Choose brushing your teeth, peeling the vegetables, walking the dog, going for a swim, washing your hands, reading a journal, saying hello to your colleagues. Practise keeping your attention on that activity for two minutes *every* time you do it. Look your colleagues in the eye (if appropriate) when you greet them, stand still and wait for their reply, smile and create time for 15 seconds. Repeat it every day, be fully present in the connection you have with them. Notice how you feel when you do.

As you practise, resist the temptation to criticise and judge yourself when your attention wanders. It's normal and expected that your attention will drift. Peeling the potatoes might not be the most stimulating thing you did today, but it's possibly more interesting than you think. Each time you practise directing and maintaining your attention, even on something you previously labelled as dull, you strengthen your attention muscles in just the same way as you strengthen your biceps each time you lift weights in the gym. As you repeatedly activate your neuronal pathways for attention, gradually your ability to pay attention and notice distraction will improve.

> My invitation is for you to notice what you are like when you are fully present and curious. What happens to the way you practise medicine when you are paying attention and you are fully aware? What happens to your health and wellbeing?

Professor Ellan Langer from Harvard has been studying mindfulness for nearly five decades. She says that we are naturally mindful in novel situations. Think of any new skill you have learnt or new place you arrived at, perhaps a new workplace holiday destination. Can you remember what it was like to look at this new place or activity with totally fresh eyes? You were probably accepting, curious and attentive. What were you aware of? Think of how a small child walking to the park learns about their environment if they are given the space to do it their way. They wander along as if there is all the time in the world, touching plants, looking underneath rocks and up high in the trees, asking questions, pondering, going back to take another look, even singing perhaps! They are open, present, interested, and curious.

These are the ideal conditions for learning. Is this how you practise medicine each day? Is this how you look after your own needs each day? Are you willing to learn about your own interior with this level of interest?

Obviously, you cannot wander through your clinic or hospital all day long like a curious young child, but you can choose one thing each day to bring your full focus to and practise. Why not practise mindfully walking from your car to your house each day – keep your mind fully on the act of walking for two minutes every day. Now you are practising mindfulness.

> **Training your attentional capacity and your awareness is the same as every other skill you have ever trained for: you need to practise.**

Having a coach or a teacher will help you stay on track, develop the right technique, and fine tune your new skills. Having a trusted peer or friend can also help you keep practising. Share what you are doing with someone. Create an accountability structure to support your habit change. When you start with regular, intentional mind-training practice, your own experience will provide you with the valuable feedback you need to keep going. Don't expect to be an expert after three tries, lean into feeling uncomfortable, that's the learning edge, keep training.

Start where you are, keep it simple. A single breath with a long exhalation that you pay attention to is a mindful meditation. You can try this simple breathing exercise.

## ACTIVITY 2

## A simple mindful breathing exercise

Take a piece of paper and create a page that you can log your experience on, you might like to copy this one. Each day, before the breathing practice, make a note of the state your mind and body are in. Be curious and gentle, there is no right and wrong answer. You are simply tuning in to your own internal environment, raising your awareness and paying attention.

E.g. Mind: focused, distracted, overwhelmed, happy
Body: tight, tense, relaxed, burdened, upright, cold

| Day | Body before practice | Mind Before practice | Body after practice | Mind after practice |
|---|---|---|---|---|
| E.g. | Tight | Overwhelmed | Less tight | Calm & distracted |
| 1 | | | | |
| 2 | | | | |
| 3 | | | | |
| 4 | | | | |
| 5 | | | | |
| 6 | | | | |
| 7 | | | | |

**Take a breath in through your nose for four counts. Now hold your breath for four counts. Breathe out for a count of six, a long slow exhalation, and now pause for a count of four before you take the next breath.**

Repeat this cycle two more times, but this time focus on the activity instead of the instructions. Keep your attention on the act of breathing and counting.

What did you *notice* as you practised? In other words, what were you *aware* of? Did your attention wander?

If you have never done something like this before, it's likely your attention did wander. I invite you to do this mindfulness practice every day for the next week, allow 1-2 minutes to complete the whole activity and do it at the same time of day if you can so that you start building a habit. Support your practice with this log if it's useful to you.

As you know, your nervous system and your biochemistry regulate your body, mostly automatically. There are many behaviours you engage in that either help or hinder achieving physiological equilibrium. The long slow exhalation for instance slows your heart rate improving your heart rate variability. We will look at this more in chapter 5.

After you have completed the week, take a look over the log and see what you notice, use whatever you notice as a tool to help you raise your awareness. Pay attention, use the log as the stimulus, sit quietly for a few moments to notice what your mind and body does in response to the information you have recorded, then *consciously choose* your response.

If you notice something new, sit with that for a few moments, observe your body and your internal environment, be curious and patient as you seek to understand and choose your next action (your response). If you notice something familiar to you, enquire with curiosity – as if you are a beginner in this space. Ask yourself questions like:

- Does this response serve me well? How?
- What value shows up?
- Am I living in alignment with this value that I am now aware of?

It is not necessarily so that you will change anything after this activity – you may, you may not. This exercise offers you a window, how you respond is up to you. If this exercise seems useful, keep going for another week. You can use any trigger you like, for instance if you are reading this book cover to cover, you might like to complete this simple mindfulness practice at the end of each chapter.

## 2. EMOTIONAL LITERACY

The second skill set to master for self-regulation is being literate about your emotions.

Emotional literacy means that you are able to understand the physiological sensations you experience – tingling, pain, temperature changes, etc. – as they arise in your body. Once you have identified these sensations, you can learn to recognise them as signposts to your emotions, gradually improving your ability to accurately name the emotion in real time.

> Practising naming your emotions and extending your emotional
> vocabulary is key to self-regulation.

### Mind interprets emotion

Your whole body is reading and sending signals to your brain. Your brain is interpreting these signals from the external environment and your internal environment 24/7. We refer to this process that involves your whole body as *mind.*

In recent years, neuroscience has been able to isolate networks of neurons in the human brain that are involved in attention, inattention, concentration, decision making, and so on. They have also studied neurons in the gut and heart. While we only have one brain, it seems there are neurons involved in perception, interoception, interpretation, decision making, and awareness elsewhere in our bodies, beyond our brains. This process of recognising information from our whole body is referred to as *embodied.* Awareness is a sensory experience that is embodied, rapid, and often unconscious, making it hard to explain entirely with rational, observable science.

Have you ever met someone new and had a 'gut feeling' about them? How about a sense of foreboding or anticipation that couldn't really be explained by factual data? This intuition is informed by your history, culture, education, and many other known and unknown variables. These physiological sensations and mental intuitions are described as emotions. When you feel emotional you are describing an internal process that involves your conscious and unconscious mind-body. You feel it physiologically and psychologically.

Your whole body is gathering data from the external world. This data is interacting with your existing mental templates (conscious and unconscious, including your biases and assumptions). Your brain sifts and selects what it deems important, then interprets and predicts, causing you to experience thoughts and sensations that you experience as emotions. Using the information and these emotions, your brain crafts a story to explain what is going on. Your brain is anticipating what will happen next and recognising associations with other experiences and things it 'knows' and deems to be relevant. This process serves to keep you safe in the world.

Humans have evolved to generate emotions in common ways and have shared descriptions of them, but *your* emotional experience is unique to you. It depends on your prior experiences, your templates. Which is why you can have the same experience (stimulus) as someone else but feel (respond) differently to it.

> **Your ability to notice the sensory data your body provides, to name it accurately and to understand what the emotion is signposting is referred to as your emotional literacy.**

Understanding and responding to emotions effectively is not the same as *being emotional.*

Even stoics, who value rational thinking, feel emotions. Stoics value virtue, *control* of emotions and human connection. Rather than controlling emotions, modern medicine has created a culture of avoiding emotions and has largely ignored the importance of human connection beyond establishing rapport, believing that doctors will not be able to do their work if they are emotional and connecting as humans. All humans are emotional beings, that's part of what defines us as human.

The first step in emotional intelligence is understanding emotions, a concept first described in the scientific literature by Mayer and Salovey in 1997. Their work has shown us that emotions make us smarter. Rather than get in the way of rational thought, emotions help us to shape thought. We will look more deeply at how emotions can help you raise your performance, leadership, and wellbeing in Chapter 6.

> Emotions are present in every interaction. In order to regulate yourself well, you need to be skilled in emotional management.

## How to train emotional literacy

You can improve your emotional literacy by being mindful and present to your own experience. One way to do this is to build in regular pauses and ask yourself curious questions such as those below. This curiosity is known by those in mindfulness circles as the 'beginner's mind'– consider your experience as if you have never seen or felt it before.

### Reflection

- What can I feel or notice in my body in this moment?
- What name would I give this sensation?
- Does this sensation indicate an emotion?
- Can I give the sensation a name that is an emotion?

For example, you might notice that your attention is drifting as you read. Turn toward this, notice it.

What else is happening in your body, are you physically comfortable?

Can you feel anything physiologically? (Do you need to use the bathroom? Are you hungry?)

Is there something in the room distracting you?

Can you give any of your physical sensations a name, like hungry or distracted? Can you then name an emotion, perhaps annoyed, bored, or torn between wanting to keep reading but needing to get something else done?

Start noticing your own emotional language. Be curious about your physical sensations and experiment with emotion words.

Take a look at the following page, how many of these emotions do you recognise in your life? Start including a wider range of words to describe your emotional life; grow your emotional literacy. As you improve your accuracy describing your own emotional experience, you will also become more skilled at recognising emotions in others. This will help you in all your relationships, improving your influence, performance, teamwork, results and sense of belonging. This increasing accuracy will help you maintain your balance and stay regulated, making you much more effective.

Amazement Alienation Defeat
Humiliation Embarrassment Dejection
Insecurity Isolation Regret Guilt
Sympathy Affection Caring Compassion
Love Enthusiasm Pride
Desire Zest Relief Eagerness
Delight Optimism Elation
Enjoyment Rapture Pleasure
Disgust Nervousness Worry Panic
Envy Anxiety Bitterness
Satisfaction Grief Tenderness
Euphoria Rage Sentimentality
Amusement Joy Grumpiness
Contempt
Frustration Irritation
Surprise Gladness Torment
Loathing Triumph
Happiness Spite Alarm Thrill

## Compartmentalising as a regulation strategy

Perhaps now you are saying that you don't want to pay attention to what you are seeing at work, that some of the human suffering you witness is better forgotten. Perhaps you are looking for a switch so you can turn your mind and emotions off, more than a way to tune into them.

Medical training has probably taught you to separate or compartmentalise your emotions, to leave them at the door in the name of professionalism. If you are a surgeon about to drill into someone's bone or saw open their chest, this may be a useful strategy. Many surgeons have told me it's essential, no less.

Compartmentalising your experiences is a suppression response to your thoughts and emotions. The problem with suppression of psychological and emotional events is that they can cause harm to you in the longer term without you realising it's happening. When you do become aware there is a problem, it's often too late.

Suppression is a fear-based strategy. It's as if each adverse or distressing event is a wild animal and the only strategy you have for managing it is by locking it in the bathroom of your house. The problem is, there may be many more wild animals that you need to lock down. Each time you have a potentially distressing event, you toss another wild animal into the bathroom. Gradually, your bathroom fills up with wild animals.

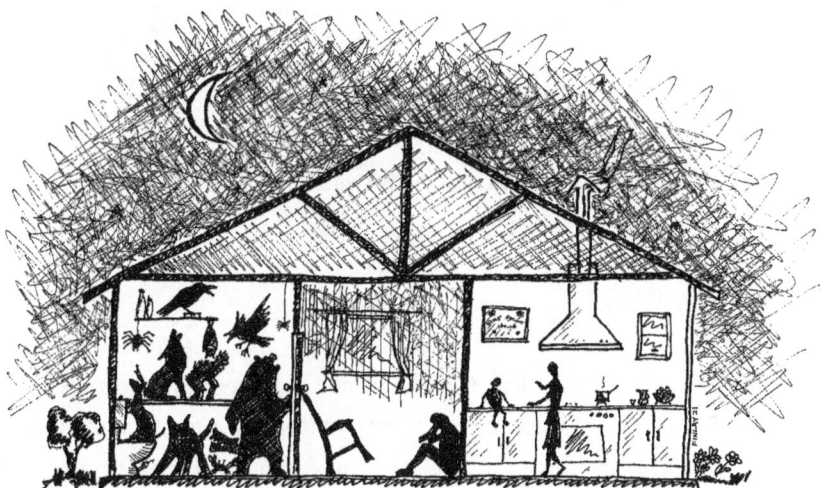

Over time as it gets more crowded in there, the animals who are eager to get some space start pushing on the door. Even though you fortify the door with furniture and locks, occasionally you have to open the door to throw another wild animal in. Every time feels more risky, perhaps there will be no more room, perhaps one will get out. You use more and more of your physical resources to keep them contained and more of your psychological resources worrying about keeping them contained. Sometimes they settle and you forget about them, but you can never truly relax, they are in your house after all. You can't unknow what you know.

> Compartmentalising has a place as a safety response that is helpful in the short term.

Compartmentalising your emotions is an effective short-term tool. If it is your only tool, you are incredibly limited in your ability to respond to the array of emotions working in medicine can elicit. It might allow you to do the work of surgery, but does it facilitate collaboration with your team? Over the longer term, it is a limiting strategy because of the energy required to maintain suppressing your thoughts and emotions. You can end up depleted because you are using your energy to contain these unresolved past experiences.

> Meeting your experiences with compassion and mindfulness is a growth and learning strategy that can help you integrate your experiences and keep you moving forward with energy and agency.

## 3. SELF-AWARENESS

There is one more skill set to master in order to regulate yourself effectively, and that is self-awareness. Self-awareness means continuously noticing what you are thinking, feeling, and doing, and remembering that there is a great deal outside your conscious knowing.

This means you recognise that:

- your perception is only one possible version of reality
- you have biases and assumptions operating that you may or may not be aware of in the moment
- you can pause and choose your response rather than reacting habitually.

> We often need to enlist the help of others to raise our awareness to our own biases. They are called blind spots for a reason – we can't see them ourselves. Unconscious bias operates in every human.

### Unconscious bias and assumption

You learnt your biases and assumptions unconsciously from the world around you simply by being immersed in it. They are built on associations and operate as short cuts (heuristics) for your brain. Although they direct your behaviour, you are mostly oblivious to their existence; they are implicit. Remembering that will help you stay more open and curious, less reactive, and more regulated.

Your biases and assumptions are active 24/7 and most of the time they are not subject to any fact checking. They may not be founded in any evidence at all. They exist to help you manage the overwhelming amount of data in the environment – they are short cuts designed to help you understand the world. The problem with these short cuts is that they narrow your field of vision, then you use these cognitive templates as if they are true without ever revising or questioning their ongoing validity. Biases create cognitive rigidity, lulling you into routine and autopilot and reducing your capacity for creative problem solving. Which is fine for standard procedure, but not for complex or changing conditions.

It's like swimming out to sea easily with an undercurrent. You may not be aware of the current, you may assume that you are an excellent swimmer, or that you are really at ease in the water. It's only when you turn around to swim back and realise how much more effort is involved that you understand you didn't have all of the information when you were swimming out. As you struggle without much progress, your awareness changes and you realise that your swimming ability hasn't changed at all, there was something else operating outside of your awareness, an undercurrent.

Understanding that bias exists in you enables you to account for it. As a result, you have a more open mind, ask more curious questions, value the various perspectives of your colleagues more, and accept your own mistakes.

> **We need to acknowledge bias so that we can take steps to mitigate the problems it creates. Mindfully and skilfully accounting for bias is an important part of self-regulation.**

Here's a simple example. Biases develop because of what we hear and see in the world. Often, they were laid down at a young age. If you grew up in a family of people who disliked eating fish, you may hold a bias against eating fish your whole life, believing you don't like it without ever even tasting it.

Let's say you go out for dinner with your new partner. You really want to impress them, and they love seafood and want to try out the new seafood restaurant. Suddenly you become aware of your unfounded bias against eating fish.

Your partner suggests the seafood restaurant and you instantly react with "I hate fish". This is an automated response arising from what psychologists call cognitive rigidity, an existing template that might also be described as limited perception or is often colloquially called black and white thinking. It is much more likely to happen under stress (remember HALLTSS) or when you perceive a threat, consciously or unconsciously.

This way of understanding the world limits your problem-solving capacity, your creativity and your acceptance and inclusion of other people and ideas. If your own rigid thinking is challenged or threatened, you are likely to double down, entrenching your narrow perception and belief.

In this example, an argument could ensue with each partner arguing vigorously for their restaurant of choice. It could even be your first argument – over something trivial, all directed by your autopilot, fear-based protection mechanisms. In this state, you have lost your ability for insight. Instead of regulating yourself in the complex changing environment, your stress response is activated, effectively taking your prefrontal cortex offline.

**Let's try that again**

You have been practising your regulation skills, and so you notice at the mention of the seafood restaurant that you feel resistant and uncomfortable. As you pause to register this feeling and name the emotion, you activate your curiosity and realise that you have never tried fish, and that your objection to it is limiting your experience. You wonder what fish tastes like, maybe you wonder if you will be allergic to it.

You are aware of your internal environment, and you are consciously managing it in service of something that is important to you – your new relationship. You can consciously choose your response: instead of reacting with something like "I hate fish", you regulate yourself and stay connected with your partner.

Awareness is the key to your active choice. You might still decide not to go to the seafood restaurant, but you don't end up in a fight defending a position that you don't even know if you care about.

## *Compartmentalising "Others"*

Unconscious biases and assumptions exist about gender, sexual orientation, heritage, education, place, values, and any other feature of a person that we might deem to be different to ourselves. When we compartmentalise another person as "other" we implicitly say they are not like us, they are set apart from us, and we are at risk of objectifying them.

> When we "other" someone, we behave differently towards them.

This can be described as your *in group* and *out group*. Us humans are more empathic to those we consider to be in our *in group* than to those in our *out group,* but we are not necessarily conscious of who we regard to be in or out. We will return to this again in Chapter 7 as it relates deeply to empathy. Without awareness, you fail to recognise how differently you relate to other people. When this is happening, your state and your biases are unconscious, and regulation is random at best. Even worse, your behaviour is directed by rigid unconscious autopilot patterns that are discriminating.

Research has demonstrated that black-skinned patients have received less pain medication because of an implicit belief that they can handle more pain than white-skinned people. There is no biological evidence that black people collectively have a higher pain threshold than others or that they are unable to determine when they are in pain and so should not be believed by their healthcare providers. But there is plenty of scholarly research to show the practice is real and common across medicine.

As a result of this biased assumption, black patients have received suboptimal care for their pain from white doctors, not because this was the doctors' intention, but because it was an unconscious bias. We are blind to our blind spots.

The more you understand this, the more you can accept help from others so that you can provide optimal care to your patients without having to get upset, defensive or reactive in your responses. It's not personal, it's not a deficiency in you, we all have unconscious biases. You cannot counter them until you know about them and, by their very nature, they are hard to know about. Be proactive in discovering them and welcome the help of others to find them so you can keep raising your awareness.

> Remember, your brain loves automation because it's efficient, but that doesn't necessarily make it effective in complex human interactions.

The benefits of raising your awareness for self-regulation are best demonstrated with some examples. The following stories are all ones that doctors have shared with me about how raising their awareness to their own implicit bias has helped them self-regulate.

Story 1 *"As a woman of colour, I have experienced a lot of bias in my career progression. My seniors have told me lots of times that* they underestimated me until they saw my work. That has been really challenging to hear, because they haven't given me opportunity to demonstrate my work! I have watched people, white males, junior to me in terms of experience, be given opportunities in preference, which has made me frustrated and angry. I've even been left thinking it's hopeless, I may as well leave medicine. Recognising that unconscious bias has played a role has helped me move past these situations and stay focused on my goals and maintaining my voice. It has also given me a language to call out these biases on behalf of others, now that I am in a senior role. There is no such thing as merit in medicine, but remembering that everyone is biased helps me stay calm when I really want to raise the roof about women of colour being treated unfairly. Because in fact, I am making more headway for them by keeping my cool."*

Story 2 *"As an anaesthetist, I am often put off and frustrated by patients with a high BMI. Recently though, someone in my* family who is overweight had an operation. I was thinking about them at the time of their surgery and noticed I was more forgiving of their weight than I would be of my own overweight patients. I am now aware of a strong bias I have had about people who are overweight and how I have communicated differently with them than my other patients. I used to feel really agitated and annoyed in surgeries with overweight patients; now I am more relaxed and I notice that my attention is actually better. I think of these people as suffering instead of lazy, and I am kinder to them in the pre-op conversation, which I like and they seem to too."*

Story 3 *"I realised I had a bias when I watched a health play and saw a patient be rude to a nurse in the play based on her* country of birth. It was really upsetting watching that play. I went back to work and spoke with my nursing colleagues about their cultures and learnt a lot from them, they were happy to help me learn. We are a much more effective team now. Once I saw this bias in myself, I started seeing it everywhere unfortunately. I no longer let any patients get away with racial commentary on the ward. I'm much more active, I was a bystander before, I just didn't understand how hurtful doing nothing was. Now I get angry at seeing my colleagues* *treated that way, I have more emotion about it, but it's ok because I know what to do with it. I try to remember it is an opportunity to help the patient learn something. I'm learning to name it, and asking others to help keep me steady."*

We all want to connect and belong, but unconscious bias is in us all and so we make mistakes. You don't know what you don't know. You do not respond to everyone in the same way. Open conversation and respectful curiosity that is culturally sensitive might make you feel vulnerable because you might hear some feedback that is uncomfortable. These conversations can show you what you can't see by yourself, and they can build trust. Self-regulation doesn't mean you stop feeling emotions, it means you are more skilled at managing them.

> **Like every other human being, you need conscious practices and other trusted people to help you see your own blind spots.**

When you bring your mindfulness, emotional literacy, and courage to the conversation, you can grow trusting relationships that will help you uncover some of your biases. Then you can actively choose how you want to behave and understand what you really believe and value. When your self-regulation skills are strong, you can lean into all sorts of experiences with more confidence.

When trust is high, your sense of psychological safety is high. In these circumstances, you are able to learn, to be vulnerable, to receive feedback and to integrate what you learn about your blind spots. You are able to raise your awareness and improve your regulation in relationships with other people.

### How to use your raised awareness to regulate and connect

To be open to learning about your unconscious biases creates a feeling of vulnerability for most people. Think carefully about who you trust and start small.

Give one person permission to share what they observe in you over time. It doesn't even have to be at work, ask your best friend or someone in your family if they are willing to talk about these ideas with you. You could start by reflecting together on something you have reacted to in the media.

Having a strong emotional response towards something is a good indicator that you either care a lot or you are confused by something. Start there. To grow and develop, to stretch outside your existing cognitive templates and your comfort zone and into your learning edge, you need trust, you need to feel safe. Look for the people you trust and when they share what they have noticed with you, thank them and take their words as a very precious gift. You don't have to accept or agree with everything you receive, accept the idea that there may be something outside your awareness that you could learn about and intentionally reflect on it.

> Get comfortable with being uncomfortable; you are not looking to be endorsed, you are looking to gain insight.

In actively seeking to understand, in acknowledging your gaps and your biases, you build trust and connection with others. Connection is the balm that soothes grief, trauma, mental illness, and burnout.

> Your mindfulness skills will help you notice your own reactive behaviours and to listen openly when others offer you feedback about bias. Your emotional regulation skills will help you sit with and then lean toward this feedback rather than avoid or reject it outright.

## ACTIVITY 3

### Try this – unearthing your biases by practising *Just Like Me*

Another way to connect with people, especially those outside of your usual experience, is to practise saying *just like me* to yourself. This practice is founded in the idea that all humans are seeking to be happy and to relieve their suffering.

If you meet a *heartsink* patient or a person who you have previously thought of as a *drug seeker*, instead of describing them to yourself in this disappointed or dismissive tone, remind yourself that at least in this essential human way you are alike. They too are seeking happiness and relief from suffering in perhaps the only way they know how, they are *just like you* in this respect.

If you notice your internal resistance when you say this to yourself regarding another person, you have probably unearthed one of your biases. If your own internal voice reacts with *no they're not anything like me*, or *I'm nothing like them,* get curious. What is your resistance about? Saying *just like me* to yourself increases your capacity for compassion. One of the important components of compassion is empathy. When you are empathic with another person, you are less likely to "other" them and make negatively bias decisions about them.

Run your own experiment, say *just like me* to yourself for a few days at work, be curious about your internal reactions – thoughts and emotions. Write them down and reflect on them in your journal or with your trusted person. Be open to learn and practise your new regulation skills as you go.

Turning towards your biases and assumptions opens the doorway to self-awareness and growth.

> **You will not improve your regulation, balance, or agency by ignoring your biases or pretending you don't have any. Why not use all of you to thrive!**

## SUMMARY

Regulating yourself well is a skill that can give you confidence and help you respond effectively to your experiences. It will help you be less reactive, but it is not a guarantee of calm waters forever. Life will keep happening, surprising you and testing your resilience, triggering emotions and challenging your capacity. That's what a rich full life looks like, even without a medical career.

Clarity of mind achieved through good sleep and mindfulness skills, emotional literacy and self-awareness (that includes understanding you are biased), are the tools you need to maintain your balance and activate your own personal agency. Once you have learnt to regulate yourself effectively, you may find that you have freed up some energy.

It's a good opportunity then to reflect on what's important to you so that you can direct this energy for maximum benefit. In the next chapter, we will explore what really matters most to you.

### Actions to improve your regulatory skills

1.  Attend to your sleep. Aim for 7-9 hours of sleep every 24 hours. Get some help to improve or redesign your sleep.
2.  Complete the activity on page 57: Envisage your best life and start *noticing* what you are doing.
3.  Start a journal or notebook where you can write what you notice down as you do the activities in this book.
4.  Notice your breath. Regularly pause and extend your exhalation. Try the breathing exercise on page 66.
5.  Practise mindfulness, improving your attention and your awareness and creating choice. Find a coach, teacher, or peer group who can help you hone your mindfulness skills.
6.  Practise naming your body's sensations and the emotions they signpost.
7.  Expand your emotions vocabulary, practise out loud with intention using the list on page 72.

8. Remember you have biases that are not necessarily true or useful but are part of being human.
9. Invite one other person to reflect on unconscious bias with you and start an ongoing conversation, giving them permission to share what they have noticed in your behaviour.
10. Your biases cause you to objectify others. Look inside yourself with curiosity first and practise saying "just like me" when you notice you are "othering" another person.

# 4 KNOW YOURSELF

*"In any given moment we have two options: to step
forward into growth or to step back into safety."*
— *Abraham Maslow, Psychologist*

Many of our daily activities happen by default, they are simply habitual, like travelling to work and eating. Do you remember what your son was talking about with you this morning, or was your attention somewhere else? How much of your time and energy, your attention, is used up on things you can't remember?

Each day, you go out into the world on autopilot – drinking coffee, navigating complex relationships, consulting, and making differential diagnoses. Some of these activities are momentary, you don't even remember them, and some are core to your identity if you stop and think about it, but you probably never do.

Are you paying attention to the things that really matter to you, or have you somehow been programmed to do what everyone else wants? What is it *you* love to do?

In this chapter I invite you to come into intimacy with yourself and your inner experience. Get up close with what matters to you, recognise your uniqueness, and step outside of what medicine has trained you to do and be. Inquire with love, kindness, and curiosity into what brings you joy, what inspires you, what **you need** to flourish as a doctor and in life. That's when your patients will have the best chance to experience excellent healthcare from you.

> This chapter is your opportunity to reconnect,
> remember and reimagine yourself.

## WHY DOES KNOWING YOURSELF MATTER?

As described in Chapter 3, what we pay attention to and are aware of is selective. Once you raise your self-awareness to this selective attention, you can be more proactive about your attention choices. As you start to notice different things, new opportunities come into your awareness and can change your life. Until then, what you are aware of and pay attention to is guided by your unconscious biases. When you consciously and actively tune in with genuine curiosity, you can start to discover what you *really* believe in and what you truly value.

Once you know what you value and have challenged what you believe, you have some powerful anchors to direct your attention, giving your life more meaning and simplicity. This is a life on purpose rather than a life on autopilot.

> Your altered internal experience will change how you relate to
> your external environment. This is empowering and improves your
> efficacy in life and work.

## ACTIVITY 4

Here's a mini audit for you to take stock of how you are living your life day to day. Take another look at Activity 1 in Chapter 3 (page 57). Answer these five questions as honestly as you can. Adjust your table as you discover what you need.

1. What activities matter to you most?
2. How often are you giving them your *best* energy, effort and attention?
3. Do you consciously prioritise them every day?

4. Could others watching you tell that these are your most important activities?

5. When do you feel completely in flow, joyful, at ease?

Is there a gap between how you answered the questions and what is really happening in your life? Do your answers provoke any insights for you about what you believe or value? What action would you like to take if you could? Write these down too.

For better or worse, your sense of purpose, beliefs, and values guide your attention and awareness in a continuous feedback loop that is largely unconscious. This process can help you or limit you depending on how attuned you are to your own inner world. As your more intimate sense of self is established, you can respond more effectively to your own needs, keeping you balanced and helping you to thrive.

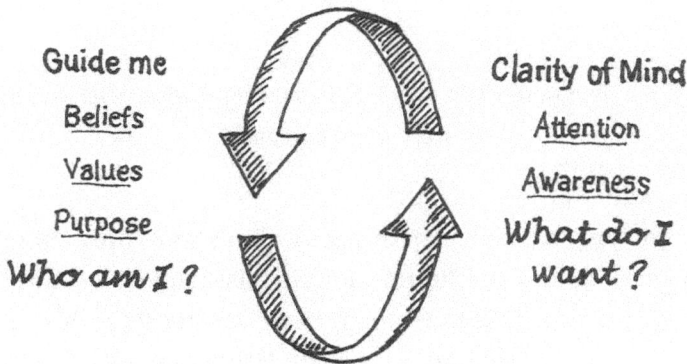

Guide me
Beliefs
Values
Purpose
Who am I ?

Clarity of Mind
Attention
Awareness
What do I
want ?

## HOW TO BUILD YOUR SELF-AWARENESS

Let's explore four factors that support your behaviour whether you are conscious of them or not. As you answered the questions above, you may have uncovered some of your motivators, making them more explicit or conscious. As you work through this chapter, practise what you learnt in Chapter 3 to regulate yourself. Use your body, breath, emotional literacy, and awareness of bias to stabilise yourself as you do the activities and reflect on the ideas. This is an opportunity to be intimate with your inner landscape, especially your 'what' and your 'why'.

To get you reacquainted with yourself, we are going to explore these four factors:

1.  Your meaning and purpose
2.  Your beliefs
3.  What you value
4.  Your sense of self.

## MEANING AND PURPOSE

*"He who has a why to live can bear almost any how."*
*— Fred Nietzsche.*

> What is your purpose in your life? In medicine? What gives you the greatest sense of meaning?

These are big questions; many people don't know the answers. If you don't know, work through the questions in this chapter with curiosity and patience. Bring some kindness to yourself and consider this process to be lifelong work. You are a complex, wonderful human being with many possibilities inside you. Explicitly naming what brings you meaning can help you create the life you want – a life lived on purpose.

If you do not know *why* you are giving your energy to medicine, it is much harder to sustain the effort involved in doing this work which asks so much of you (and your family). Give some thought to what you need to support yourself in this state of not knowing. It's time well spent as you reset and rediscover who you are, what you need and how you might go forward in a way that will bring meaning and fulfilment into your life.

Once you can articulate your *why*, everything becomes personal – you feel connected to it, you can take ownership and feel engaged and energised by it. Knowing what's important to you helps you find your *how*, your way to keep progressing, when you experience a setback. Having clarity of mind about your why doesn't mean everything is suddenly easy but it does mean you have an anchor in rough conditions and a sense of direction.

> **When you know what you care about, what is meaningful to you, what is aligned to your values, you have a much higher likelihood of enjoying your work.**

# Janice's Story

*Janice is a paediatrician I have known for many years. She came to me in tears, overwhelmed with the needs of her patients and the high level of support some of their parents needed. In that moment of overwhelm she said, "It's all too hard, it's too much effort. It doesn't matter how much effort I make, it's not enough. These families have so much difficulty in their lives."*

*We talked about what was important to her in her work, essentially what gets her out of bed in the morning. Thinking back to why she trained to be a paediatrician in the first place, she told me about a time during her intern year when a child had died of complications. That had always stayed with her. She went on to tell me how remembering that little boy had helped her work through some of the very difficult family interactions she'd had during her advanced training and since.*

*By remembering this and other stories, Janice reconnected with her previous value-based decisions to always help the families she worked with feel seen and heard. Her belief that everyone deserves access to great healthcare grounded her. We talked about effort, reframing and exploring where else Janice's energy went. How did she decide what to give her effort to?*

*Using this new understanding of her purpose, we reviewed what she believed about her own wellbeing and boundaries. She set guidelines for herself and developed a language to enhance her internal response to distressed parents*

*of the children she works with. She decided that she did want to keep giving*
*her effort to her patients and their families.*

Purpose gives you a frame of reference that helps you understand what is happening and helps you make decisions that are right for you. This internal scaffold fortifies your regulation ability and helps to keep you balanced even while you work with the complexities of healthcare and the vagaries of life.

> Consider your external environment after you understand your internal needs; what really gives you purpose and meaning?

I have partnered with many independent pathway doctors from overseas as their coach. Some of these doctors sit exams that will allow them to practise as rural generalists multiple times before they fellow. These persistent doctors offer a vivid example of purposeful action based on personal meaning. For them, passing their exams means independence, freedom, and future security. Their purpose is often about creating opportunity for their family, which is deeply meaningful. They have uprooted their whole lives and moved to a new country.

This clarity and deeply held meaning is exactly what fuels their determination. Although they feel vulnerable, their confidence is tested. They study for years, but these doctors sustain their effort by focusing on a better future for the people they love. That's what they really care about in the moments when it all feels too hard.

The system is problematic and challenging for these doctors, but there is a clear purpose that keeps them focused, that directs their actions in line with what is meaningful. Their clear purpose is their most potent motivator. When they give their energy to the systemic challenges, there is little to be gained except frustration, resentment, dysregulation, and more risk of failure. It is a distraction and a barrier to what really matters. The external environment is tough and out of their control. They focus their energy and mind internally where they have some control. They activate their personal agency.

> The aim here is not to paint some unattainable fantasy life. The aim is to understand what it is you really want in your life so that you have some capacity to create it.

Shanafelt et al found that when doctors in corporate clinics and big hospitals are able to spend 20% of their work time doing what they love, work that is personally meaningful to them, then they are willing to spend the other 80% of their work time engaged in work the organisation needs them to do.

In other words, doctors recognise they will need to do a range of work and they will not necessarily enjoy it all. As long as there is a portion that is fulfilling for you, then you have sustainability and are likely to remain engaged in your work. Your 20% might be research, working in a community clinic, or being on a committee whose purpose you value.

What's your 20% at work that you love? What work were you doing when it felt like the time flew by or you were in the zone, in flow?

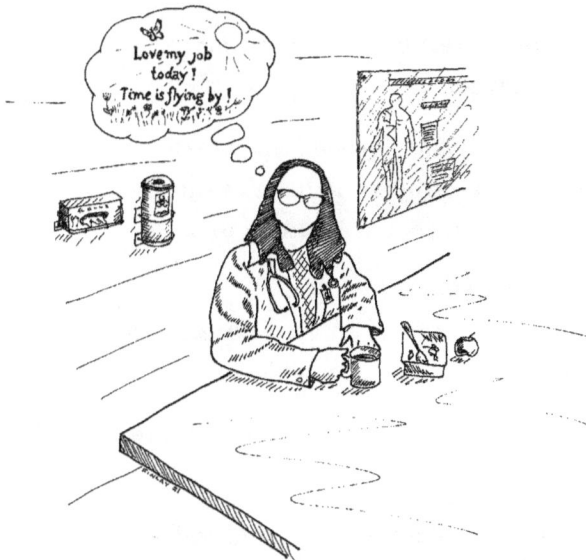

## HOW TO FIND YOUR MEANING

Focusing on your **intention** can be more helpful than focusing on the outcome when you are thinking about your meaning. Making your intentions explicit directs your attention toward what gives you meaning. Consider the following:

- What is your intention as a doctor?
- What action are you taking to demonstrate your intention, to bring it to life?
- What do you want to be known for?

> When you understand what you want, you can set about creating the right environment and developing the skills you need to achieve it.

You can ask yourself about your intention any time, and for any time frame or activity. You can be general or specific with your intention. Intention questions are about how you want to behave, what you want to experience, what you want to tune into. Intentions direct and guide your efforts and attention.

**Below are some examples of intentions.**
**General - Go large:**

*What is my intention for my medical career?*
My intention is to learn how to balance the art and science of medicine well, giving equal attention to both.

*What is my intention this year?*
My intention this year is to improve my emotional literacy through conscious and overt practice.

These intentions can be big and bold. Here are a couple more examples:

- My intention is to always be a kind colleague.
- My intention is to prioritise the patient's goals.

**Specific - Go small:**

*What is my intention for this next patient encounter?*
My intention is not to interrupt for the first three minutes while the patient tells me their story.

*What is my intention for the next 10 minutes?*
My intention is to practise mindfulness by keeping my full attention on reading this journal article.

These intentions can be tiny and very specific, keeping us focused and on task. Here are some more examples:

- My intention is to turn my phone off for the next 30 minutes.
- My intention is to attend this meeting with compassion, I know everyone is tired.

Understanding what brings you meaning and what feels purposeful allows you to tell others what you need and how you can work together, building relationships and creating environments that help you thrive. Knowing your purpose helps you act consistently with integrity and to orient yourself in times of challenge. Your *why* anchors you so you can steady your own course, improving your ability to regulate yourself. This creates a feeling of agency and empowerment, so you can start believing in your own power to create the life you want.

> Imagine relying on a clear vision of what your life is all about. Knowing intimately and explicitly why you do what you do. Then applying your technical competency and clinical skills with intention to your meaning.

Vicky's Story

*Vicky is an obstetrician and gynaecologist who has worked in a developing country for many years. Her work has reduced the mortality rate of mothers and babies in childbirth, a wonderful outcome. The impact of her work is felt throughout the whole community. People are no longer so downtrodden and frightened about childbirth, and there is much less grief caused by the loss of mothers and babies.*

*It is not easy living in this poor community, but Vicky loves it. She deeply believes her work builds a stronger community and improves everyone's quality of life; it is this that gives her meaning. She was struggling with communicating her life choices to the people she loves back in Australia. She often felt like she was defending herself, and felt pressure to conform to expectations about her career in medicine.*

*In our coaching sessions, Vicky was able to understand herself and why she made the bold choices that she has. She is living on purpose. Her intention to help this community and to lift their quality of life through better healthcare keeps her going when she wonders why she isn't living a life of physical comfort back in Australia. Instead of reacting to other's questions about when she would return home or progress her career, she developed tools to maintain her belief no matter their opinions. As a result, she felt more settled in her clarity and more accepting of herself.*

Meaning making often extends beyond the individual. This human capacity to think of the greater good is significant for people in hard times like grief. Think of all the causes that are born out of people's adverse lived experiences. When there doesn't seem to be a clear purpose for yourself, think about the people around you and see what you would intend for them. Clarify your why by looking at the bigger picture – is there a greater good that inspires you?

## BELIEFS

Your beliefs have come from your culture, history, education, parents, other people around you, and from the media. They show up as thoughts repeating in your mind, reinforcing what you believe about the world and yourself, whether they are objectively true or not.

Here are a couple of examples:

- *I'm not good enough, I'll never get on the training program.*
- *Women are not capable of working as surgeons.*

- *White people are not biased against people of colour, I'm not racist.*
- *I need my phone with me at all times.*

> **A belief is something we 'know' to be true even though we cannot necessarily prove it.**

Without any conscious effort on your part, you have selectively paid attention to information in the world (data) that has supported your beliefs, whether they are objectively true or not, in a self-perpetuating cycle. You probably know this as confirmation bias. You have consciously noticed the supporting data and unconsciously missed, or unintentionally ignored, the contrary data.

Without awareness, your beliefs become your truth – your operating system – and they can last way beyond their use by dates unless you take an active interest.

## ACTIVITY 5

### What I know so far

Imagine we are in a coaching conversation and I am asking you these actual questions. Say the answers out loud or write them down. If you want to amplify your coaching experience, answer the questions out loud in front of the mirror and write down what seems important, new or confusing, so you can come back to it another day and reflect some more.

Think about your own journey through medicine to date. What is it that you *believe* that has you committing so much time and energy to medicine year on year?

1. What do you believe about yourself as a doctor?
2. Do you believe that you are able to be the kind of doctor you want to be?
3. Does this kind of doctoring give your life meaning?

4. What enables you to be the doctor you envisage?
5. What stops you from becoming that doctor?
6. What do you believe about medicine more broadly?

Resist the temptation to blame external forces like *the system or the culture*, avoid motherhood statements like, *well I'm a woman...* dig deep into your own heart.

**What is it that you believe to be true about yourself as a doctor?**

Few people arrive at university and study medicine accidentally. Cast your mind back a few years now:

1. What brought you to medicine in the first place?
2. Were you free to choose or were you meeting someone else's expectation when you started studying medicine?
3. Was it your first preference, the life you dreamed of?
4. What was that dream or goal driving the younger you?
5. Write your answers in the words your younger self would have used.
6. What were you aspiring to?
7. What did you believe you were doing back then?

What comes up when you make space for this work is not always what you have predicted in your busy habitual medical life. Now that you have reminded yourself about how this medical journey began and taken a quick audit of your experience so far, what still resonates with you?

1. What have you remembered as you've answered these questions?
2. What has medicine and life more broadly taught you?
3. What else has emerged for you?
4. Have you shifted away from those original beliefs, or do they still guide your decisions about your life?

Take a few minutes now and write yourself a list of the principles guiding your life. These are your beliefs. We'll call this 'What I know so far'. Write as many principles or guiding rules, **beliefs,** as you are aware of.

1.  What is it that you actually believe? Write your beliefs in the first column. Keep writing until you cannot think of anything else. See the example on p. 99 to help with brainstorming.
2.  Go through your list of beliefs and make some notes about each one. Include how active this idea currently is in your life, any emotional response that accompanies the belief and any action that becomes obvious to you.
3.  As well as writing down your beliefs, say them out loud to yourself using your own name.

Vicky, our O&G doctor working overseas, might say to herself, "Vicky believes that the wellbeing of mothers and their babies lifts the whole community's wellbeing and spirit".

Notice how you feel as you say and hear yourself voicing your belief out loud. Notice your body, whether you feel uncomfortable or very relaxed. Your body is telling you something. If you are questioning something you hear, sit with that for a while, lean into the confusion or the resistance you feel. Just because you believed something before doesn't mean you have to keep it. Does it still serve you? Does it still seem true to you, or have you learnt important information that now means letting that belief go or giving it a bit more nuance?

4.  Do you notice any gaps between what you believe and how you behave?
5.  Now assess which of your beliefs are alive in your medical practice today. Which ones you have neglected? Which ones no longer seem relevant now they are in black and white on the page? You can start making a plan if something seems obvious to you. Perhaps you need to tell someone you trust and discuss what action to take. Perhaps you need to learn some more about something you have uncovered.

| | Belief | How important is it now? | Emotions I feel about this | Actions I need to take |
|---|---|---|---|---|
| 1 | | | | |
| 2 | | | | |
| 3 | | | | |
| 4 | | | | |
| 5 | | | | |
| 6 | | | | |
| 7 | | | | |
| 8 | | | | |
| 9 | | | | |
| 10 | | | | |

| What I know so far – belief (my truth) | Value, emotion that arises | How important? Alive, neglected, no longer relevant, useful / not useful? | Action |
|---|---|---|---|
| People can and do change | Adults continue to grow and develop | Yes alive | Don't write people off |
| I love working in medicine | I feel useful, joyful, like I can help | Yes useful | Keep going |
| I am not able to work in this hospital, maybe I'm not cut out to be a doctor | Confused, medicine is ruthless, only men get promoted here | Alive<br>Not useful - I worked hard to be a doctor. | Coaching<br>Mentor<br>Discuss with friend |
| To get into the training program I have to say yes to whatever they ask me to do or someone else will do it and I will miss out | I have to sacrifice my own health to make it in medicine<br>I worked too hard to miss this opportunity<br>Value is something about deserving or fairness | Not useful, doing me harm, don't know what other options I have | Career counselling |
| I wanted to be a teacher | I had to do what my father wanted, angry | No longer relevant<br>Found a way to be a teaching doctor | |

> Let's unearth your beliefs so you can reflect on how they do or do not serve you. Then you can consciously and intentionally choose your response.

This work is whole of life work. Maintain your curiosity and value your own personal development, be your own best friend for fulfilment, balance, and connection. Perhaps it all depends on what you believe!

**Let's look at two examples of how this works.**

## Joanne's Story

*Joanne was working as a registrar in a regional hospital. She liked working in the country; there were lots of opportunities for her to expand her skills that she might not have had in a big city hospital. Her supervisor gave her constructive feedback and she passed her recent physician clinical exams. Jo was excited that the prospect of fellowship was so close now. Still, there was a persistent voice inside her head that was convinced that any day now she would be shown up as not good enough to be a doctor. No matter how hard she worked, how much positive feedback she received, or how successful she seemed, she continued to believe that she wasn't good enough. The thought of being a consultant terrified her more and more the closer she got.*

*One day she shared her fears with her supervisor, David. He had always been encouraging and she trusted him. He recognised her fear and named it – imposter syndrome. He told Joanne that every doctor he knew had experienced this sometime in their career. He said he experienced it recently when he spoke at a conference. This helped Joanne to name her fear of being a consultant and not being good enough. She reframed these thoughts by saying to herself, "David and I share this thought; it connects us". This helped her feel safe and 'normal' (a sense of belonging). She also said to herself, "This idea keeps me on my toes and helps me be present and concentrate".*

Recognising this emotion and thought pattern meant Joanne could name her **belief**: *I'm not good enough and I'm frightened.* Naming what was happening internally gave her some relief. She learnt to manage her emotions and thoughts by calling them out to herself, sometimes she also told her colleagues it was happening. Gradually she learnt to hold some other beliefs as primary, beliefs like *I am here to serve and do the best I can for my patients*, and *I choose to be a doctor who is continually learning*.

The imposter syndrome belief – *I'm not good enough to be a consultant and someone is going to find out* – still exists, but now that Joanne is consciously aware of it and has learnt the skills she needs to manage it, she isn't derailed or undermined by it like she used to be. She is consciously choosing where to put her attention and energy. She is aware of the belief, the stories and the emotions that come with it. Her raised awareness and attention skills mean she can manage and choose. When she needs to, she reframes her stories of fear and doubt into stories of empowerment and agency.

## Brian's Story

*Brian is the medical director of a large city hospital. He has attended a meeting today with the CEO and the General Manager of People and Learning because there has been a complaint against him from a senior doctor for racism and harassment. This is not the first complaint Brian has had to answer to. He phones his good friend Peter on the way home from work. Peter is a partner at a global accounting firm and works with people from all over the world. He knows it can be lonely at the top and feels for his mate, but he has himself thought Brian to be racist sometimes when he talks about his work colleagues.*

*Brian tells Peter how angry he is and how unfair the situation is. He says this would never have happened 10 years ago to his predecessor. He claims that the junior doctors are out to get him, and the senior doctors want his job. Brian tells Peter he has to attend a course on empathy and cultural sensitivity and asks Peter, "What am I going to tell the staff I am doing? I can't say that!".*

*Brian believes he is innocent and shows little insight into what others have identified as a problem. There are serious consequences to this, both for Brian and for the people who work with him. His beliefs are hindering his growth and learning, and they are limiting his relationships.*

Attending the course may raise Brian's awareness and help him pay attention to some things that have previously been outside his awareness. If this happens, he may be able to change. If he attends the course and feels psychologically safe there, he may even transform. Equally, in one or more of his relationships (perhaps with Peter, the CEO (his boss), or the GM), someone he trusts may speak up and challenge his behaviour. We often need other people to help us see our **beliefs and our blind spots.** More than that, others can encourage us in learning how to behave once we have found these harmful beliefs, as they can be quite shocking and threatening initially.

It is normal for all humans to resist new information about ourselves, because we feel vulnerable. This is an area in which gentle coaching is particularly powerful. If you are having this experience or supporting someone who trusts you through a process of uncovering blind spots and beliefs, go gently, leave some space for processing, and see it as an ongoing conversation. Pressure and insistence from others will keep the person's stress response heightened and potentially act as a learning barrier. An initial defensive reaction may often seem final, but it is possible to learn and change.

Brian is not necessarily resistant to changing his beliefs. He needs to first become aware that they may not be serving him in useful ways. In time and with trust, he may transform his beliefs, but he will need a safe space to do the work, a growth mindset, and the intention to learn. He will also need the qualities of mindfulness. In particular curiosity, patience, and acceptance of himself and of those trying to help him develop.

> *"The man who moves mountains begins by carrying*
> *away small stones." — Confucius*

## RESPONDING TO YOUR BELIEFS BY REFRAMING THE STORIES YOU TELL YOURSELF

Your beliefs might also be called your **dominant stories.** By 'story' I mean to say a description rather than something made up. You probably don't even notice your own story making, you behave and think of your dominant story as the truth or the only description until you or someone else consciously brings your enquiring attention and awareness to it. This meta-cognition requires reflection and is important for raising self-awareness.

When you start thinking about your own thinking, you might realise the story you believe is the main story you tell yourself, or perhaps you call it the *truest* of the possible stories. Your brain likes efficiency, the most efficient way to deal with overwhelming amounts of data is to select out the data that seems most important in the context of your existing lens and build it into the existing story. As Daniel Kahneman, the Nobel laureate researcher and author of *Thinking Fast and Slow* concludes, if the story seems about right, good enough, you will accept it.

> **Your dominant story (belief) is the story with the most traction or currency in your mind, in your current context.**

Perhaps you have the most evidence for this story, or it's the most believable, or the people around you also endorse it. None of this makes it the best, the truest or the only story in any objective sense. There is little value in determining the *truest* story, better to ask yourself a question that comes from Acceptance and Commitment Therapy:

> **Even if this story is 100% true, is it serving me?**

Reviewing your beliefs will mean noticing your thoughts, just like Joanne did and Brian will need to do. Your thoughts are descriptions of the world that you tell yourself to keep track and understand the data collected by your senses and your body more generally. No more and no less. These thoughts are your stories, and they are based on your conscious and unconscious beliefs.

When you question your beliefs and see your story from a new perspective, you become aware of other possible descriptions. Then, you can reframe your experience so that it serves you better. Reframing is an incredibly useful tool to help you move forward. Hold your beliefs lightly and curiously, entertain what else might be possible.

Let's look at Joanne's imposter story for an example. Her story (belief) about being an imposter wasn't serving her well. It was creating feelings of fear. She was using lots of energy second guessing herself and it had the potential to erode the confidence of those around her. Once she reframed her imposter story to '*I choose to be a doctor who is continually learning*', she felt empowered and was then able to use her energy more effectively. Instead of getting stuck, she could progress forward.

Here are a couple more examples of how you might reframe an unhelpful belief.

*I am going to fail*    →   I need to study hard to reduce my stress and risk.

*My boss hates me*   →   I need to build relationships with more than one consultant

or

→   I need to spend more time with my supervisor and get to know her better.

> Beliefs are subject to negativity bias and unconscious bias.

Humans understand the world in stories, and there is always more than one story we can tell that is true. Your brain has a negative bias. If there is ambiguous or unclear information, your brain will err towards the negative. It is much more useful to know if your belief is serving you in some useful or helpful way than to try to prove its subjective truth value.

There are two human factors to keep in mind regarding yours and others' beliefs.

1. You are an unconsciously biased being who makes mistakes AND who can learn
2. You need other people to help you notice your beliefs and bias SO you can learn

This is a proactive, open position that allows us to notice other possible stories (beliefs), to gain perspective, and to focus on solutions rather than trying to prove any given story as true. Holding these human factors in mind will allow personal growth and learning, cooperation and collaboration, acceptance and inclusion.

> It is not useful to create a story about how bad or wrong you are.

Being able to detach from binary ideas about right and wrong and good and bad will help you to reframe your thoughts. Think of your beliefs as guiding principles that you mould as you live your life, learning what serves you best along the way. Keep tuning in with your beginner's mind. Every moment is a new opportunity to discover and learn.

Self-compassion is important while you do this work. It can be really taxing. Here's a short practice to help you centre before you go on to learn about how your values can guide you.

## ACTIVITY 6

**Try this:**
- Sit comfortably with both of your feet on the ground.
- Uncross your arms and legs, and rest your hands comfortably on your legs.
- Close your eyes or cast your gaze downwards.
- Bring your attention to your breath and observe the next three inhalations and exhalations.
- Detach from any thoughts of what you should or should not be.
- Simply breathe and feel relief, knowing nothing is required of you.
- As you open your eyes, say your own name out loud followed by '*you are enough*'.

  _____, you are enough. *I am enough.*

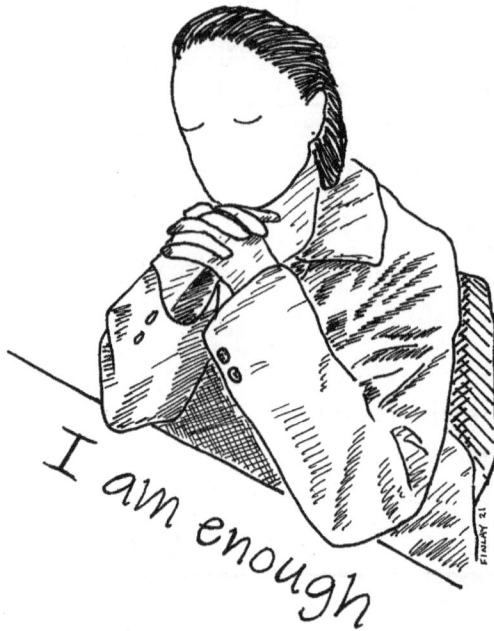

I am enough

## YOUR VALUES DESCRIBE WHAT MATTERS MOST TO YOU

Like your beliefs, your values initially come from your parents and other people around you, your culture, history, education, the media, etc., all telling you who you should be and how you should show up in the world. The word '*should*' implies obligation. As you matured, you gradually distilled your values of choice, leaving some of your childhood values behind. The values you live by in adulthood are central to how you see yourself and how you show up in the world. Your adult values are chosen by you over time and are central to your identity and core to your sense of self.

> Can you name your values and recognise how they guide your behaviour and sense of self?

Steve's Story

*In my coaching sessions with Steve, an ICU specialist, intention questions came up early. Steve was angry because some of his colleagues had sought a review of his practice after an adverse event, which is what had brought him to coaching. The review found his work and his processes to be above reproach and he was relieved, but he still felt angry. He was left wondering who to trust at work and whether he could keep working with his current colleagues. As I asked him a series of intention questions, we began to find an interesting pattern. He didn't always know the answers to what he wanted, but he was able to clearly tell me what he didn't want in his life and work.*

*Steve felt betrayed by his colleagues, some he had worked with for 12 years. In talking through all the stories he held, he discovered that what mattered most of all to him was his reputation. He had worked hard to establish it for 30 years and now believed it was significantly damaged. Steve's insight into how much he valued his reputation helped him think through what he needed going forward in order to feel safe at work, what he was willing to do or not in terms of his collegial relationships.*

*Steve did not want to stay angry, and in fact was a bit confused by his strong emotional reaction. Naming his values helped him decide what to focus on and how to behave. Ultimately, Steve's emotions dissipated, a natural occurrence that wouldn't have happened if he had suppressed his anger. He felt more in control again once he gained some clarity about what mattered the most to him – what he valued.*

Your core values are those which nourish you; those you want to live by; those which are easy to give your time and energy to. They describe what matters most to you. Values-based living is often described as being well aligned – we live with ease in this state.

> **When you bring your attention and awareness to your values, they guide you back to your purpose anchors, helping you align who you want to be with your intentions and your behaviours.**

## YOU CHOOSE YOUR VALUES AND THEN THEY MOTIVATE YOU

A little note here to help you raise your awareness and tune into your values: every time you *should* yourself, replace it with *could* and notice if your internal world shifts a little. Does your perspective and attention alter to be more open to possibilities instead of obligation? *Should* is self-talk built on a sense of obligation and duty. *Could* implies you have a choice. When you feel empowered and have agency, you are alive with possibilities and you remember that you have a choice, that *you* are in control of your decisions and therefore your life. Replace 'should' with 'could' whenever you notice it and see how you feel.

> The 'could' mindset is very different to the 'should' mindset. The 'should' mindset locks you into doing what matters to other people. When you ask 'Who *could* I be?', different possibilities arise.

Values are about who you want to *be* in the world and how you show up. For example, if you believe that integrity is important, how could you behave? You might answer, *I could be truthful and follow through on what I said I would do.* What you value guides your behaviour.

A doctor who values their work because they want to help people has quite a different frame to a doctor who became one because their parents expected them to. In the former example, the doctor is focused on helping others be well, the value might be *service*. In the latter, the doctor values being a dutiful or loyal son/daughter, the value might be *family loyalty*. Of course, you can value both, it's not necessarily either/or. I am simply demonstrating to you that your values are central to your identity, to your decisions and to how you see yourself. We cannot assume that all doctors hold the same personal values. In fact, it is this kind of assumption about other people's values that often gets in our way in relationships, creating confusion and conflict.

When you live true to your values, you feel authentic. When we judge something to be authentic, we are evaluating whether it is real, genuine or true (Beverland and Farrelly 2010). Perceptions of authenticity affect people's judgements and behaviour towards others (Smith, Newman and Dhar 2016). Your values point you toward what matters, helping you to find the activities, actions, people and habits that are the best fit for you, the ones that allow you to be your best self over time. Ultimately, other people will know you by your values and judge you by them too. It's important that you understand them if you are to know yourself.

## HOW YOU CAN IDENTIFY YOUR PERSONAL VALUES

Can you name your most important values? Most people say mention health, family, friends, or happiness. If you asked the five people closest to you what they think matters most to you, what would they say? Often others can see us more clearly than we can see ourselves.

Take another look at the ideal week you planned out in Activity 1 in Chapter 3. What did you give highest priority to? Why? What values do these activities attest to?

Where you spend your time, energy and money can point you to what you value. A note of caution though: this can be misleading, as many people spend their time, energy and money on distractions, avoiding what is truly important. An example would be staying at work for more hours than you really need to as a way of avoiding difficulties at home. Of course, you might also be staying back at work because you value hard work or duty. Or you might be driven by obligation, a default autopilot behaviour that is not at all aligned to your values and is making you unhappy and resentful. Another example is spending your time and money misusing drugs or alcohol as a means of coping or surviving. These are avoidance tactics, and distractions from what really matter.

# ACTIVITY 7

Perhaps a better way to determine your values is to think back on your best and worst times.

1.  If you have experienced an adverse or seminal event at work, how did you react?
    What was most important to you at the time?
    What seems important now?
    Did you make decisions then that you now regret? Did you make decisions that you are proud of?
    What values do you notice were guiding your decisions then and/or your reflections now?

Write whatever you notice down and keep reflecting on what matters to you.

2.  Think of the times in your life where decisions have been clear and the times where you have felt angst.
    What came to the fore as you made those decisions?

3.  If the work you have done so far in this chapter has not helped you crystalise your values, take a few moments to isolate your 10 most important values.

To help you name your values, look at the list of 50 common core values on the next page from James Clear's website. What matters most to you on this list? What defines who you are, how you think and behave? What do you put your energy into?

4.  Once you have your list of 10 values, see if you can isolate the 5 most important, the deal breakers.
    What could you live without if you really had to, and which ones are absolutely key to who you are?

5.  You can also use this online tool from the University of Western Australia to help you start articulating what your values are beyond those that medicine determines for you.
    https://www.thevaluesproject.com

Authenticity    Authority    Autonomy

Achievement    Adventure    Balance

Challenge    Boldness    Beauty

Curiosity    Community

Compassion    Competency    Determination

Citizenship    Creativity

Contribution    Friendships    Faith    Fame    Fun

Fairness    Honesty    Happiness

Humor

Justice    Growth    Loyalty

Inner Harmony    Influence    Love

Knowledge    Learning

Leadership

Kindness    Optimism

Meaningful Work    Openness

Poise    Pleasure    Respect    Religion

Reputation

Peace    Responsibility    Recognition

Popularity

Spirituality    Self-Respect    Security

Stability    Status    Success    Wealth    Service

Trustworthiness    Wisdom

If you can clearly state what you value, you have a clear blueprint that can guide your decisions authentically. This is especially useful when you are stressed and it's hard to think clearly. Together with your purpose and beliefs, your values describe the essence of you, who you are at heart.

> When your values are alive in your daily activities, you will feel at your steadiest. You will feel confident in yourself. Personal agency comes easily then too. You are aligned, have clarity of mind, and feel balanced.

Psychologist Steven Hayes, who is credited with establishing Acceptance Commitment Therapy (ACT), suggests that once you have established your values you might rightly ask yourself, *"So what?"* He is pointing to the important link between values and behaviour in being well and having a clear sense of self.

Having established your values, go a step further:

1. What are you going to stand for and be proud of in your life?
2. What **committed action** will you take to demonstrate your values?
3. How will you choose to live your values?
4. What do you need so that you can be true to yourself more often?

When you know your values and live true to them, you are more likely to experience a strong sense of purpose, meaning and fulfilment. Living authentically is easier to sustain than trying to fit into someone else's prescription because it feels like it matters. You care about it, you know why you are doing what you do. This is a highly sustainable way to live, your energy and attention is going to what you care about in a virtuous cycle.

> When there is a good fit between your values and your workplace's values, you are more likely to be engaged in your work, give discretionary effort, and to trust your colleagues.

It's not always possible to align your own meaning and values with those of your colleagues, your patients, or your workplace. Where values do not align, you are more at risk of moral injury and burnout. It is harder to derive meaning and purpose and to feel your own efficacy in an environment you don't value or one where you don't feel valued or where you cannot honour your own values.

John's Story *John worked hard as a urologist for 10 years in a large tertiary hospital. He mentored trainees, participated in various committees, and worked flexibly with his colleagues, negotiating theatre lists and sharing resources. When the director of the unit announced his retirement, John felt pressure from others within his organisation to take on the role. He did not want to apply for the director's job. He valued his time with his teenage children who would leave home soon, and he already worked 60 hours a week.*

*When the director retired, and no one was appointed to the job, John found he was the default director by virtue of his experience and time working there. No one discussed the situation with him, people just started bringing him their problems, expecting him to attend various meetings and blaming him for things that went wrong. John felt guilty and resentful. He contemplated resigning. He considered only working in the private sector and taking early retirement, even though he had previously been happy in his job. John was experiencing a values challenge through no real making of his own. What was the correct course of action?*

*If John agreed to become the director of the urology unit at his hospital even though he did not personally value being in the role, he may become resentful, working more hours, doing more administrative activities and less clinical work, and seeing less of his family. In this situation, John would have betrayed his own core value of family and as a result he is more at risk of burnout, stress, conflict, fatigue, and error. This may have negative consequences for John, his patients, his colleagues and his family.*

*Instead, if John focuses on his family values and articulates them a little more clearly, he might ask himself about his role as a father and what values he would like his children to develop. As he does this, he gives more of his mental energy and attention to his family values, raising his awareness of what's important. John may feel energised by his sense of connection with his children, and this may fortify his actions at work to draw some clearer boundaries around what he accepts from his colleagues.*

> **Betraying your values leads to harm.**

Knowing what your core values are and what innate need they meet can help you achieve your goals and therefore lead to more fulfilment. Importantly, when a values challenge arises, you are better able to resolve the way forward if you are able to articulate what you value, what you really care about.

> **Sometimes you do have to prioritise one value against another for longer- or shorter-term goals.**

If you are taking on a long-term goal like becoming a doctor or entering a training program that will take you six years or more, understanding why you are doing it is going to help you sustain your effort. It's a heck of a lot of your life you are giving over to it otherwise.

There are lots of ways to help you establish what your beliefs and values are. If these pages have been challenging for you, enlist some help. Start by sharing this experience with someone you trust, consider including a coach or a psychologist in your support team and recognise this personal development work as central to your ongoing wellbeing and performance as a doctor. Knowing yourself and what you need is central to balance, empowerment and flourishing.

> **You can use your core values to help motivate you towards your goals, they are crucial to feeling fulfilled.**

Doctors often ask me how they can motivate themselves. I use their experiences with their patients to help them think this question through. How do you motivate your patients to lose weight, stop smoking, or reduce their work hours? Do you notice that it's easier when the person really cares about it? Only one in seven people who have had a heart attack make the lifestyle changes their doctor recommends. Changing habits is difficult, even when your habit is shown to be threatening your life. It's hard to change. Finding something you really value underneath the change will help. How many times have we witnessed people lose weight when a big occasion like their wedding is on the horizon?

People say, "I just don't *feel* motivated". Motivation is an emotional state, meaning it waxes and wanes; it's fickle. Waiting for just the right motivation is a fool's game. Better to activate yourself mentally with a decision based on what you value and care about. As you take action on what is meaningful to you, your emotions will change. Relying on motivation to activate you is just too random for a high-achieving person like you.

> **You can create your own motivation and sustain it if you take the time to understand yourself, in particular your values; they are what matter to you the most.**

It's tempting to go straight to establishing goals, setting priorities, and learning about your strengths. These are all useful processes for progressing your intentions into actions, but underlying them are your beliefs and values. If you do not understand your beliefs and values, you are limited by the way they continually and unconsciously direct your attention and awareness. Slow down and do the work of understanding what drives you first.

> **Values-based action generates skills in what matters most. Confidence is the natural outcome.**

Confidence is born of action that is delivering on your intention. As you build your skills and deliver on your nominated outcomes, your confidence grows.

## YOUR ROLE OF DOCTOR IS ONLY ONE PART OF YOUR SELF

> You are not your role; your role is only one part of you.

Working in the role of doctor does not limit you from simultaneously holding many other roles. Daughter, aunty, basketball coach, triathlete, committee member, teacher, and mentor, for instance. The list is endless. Each individual role you take may show different qualities or dimensions of your *self* and none may be the same as how you would describe your whole *self*.

For most of the 20th century until now, medicine has asked doctors to keep their *self* separate from their role. *'Don't show emotion to your patients, emotions will interfere with your ability to remain calm and clear'* has been the prevailing advice. *'Keep patients at arm's length, don't share too much about yourself'* is standard advice for junior doctors.

> The way you show up in any of your roles is contextual and relative. There will be differing levels of psychological safety. As a result, you will show more or less your self in various roles.

Roles are given to us implicitly and explicitly by ourselves and by others. For example, you might assume the role of leader in a professional development workshop without anyone asking you to take it on. Others might look to you at work as if you are the leader even though you may not be formally in a role of leadership in the organisational hierarchy, like John the urologist. An implicit assignment of role that you may or may not accept. And of course you can be explicitly named in a role, such as when you are successful after applying for a job.

Roles are *socially assigned* and have within them behaviour patterns that are recognised by others. The behaviour and expectations of a role are usually described by outside forces (a job description or a college guideline, for example). These behaviours and expectations articulated by others are collectively accepted or agreed.

For example, your trainees accept that you will determine what activities they will do in their rotation that you supervise. They accept that you will assess their level of competence to work unsupervised in your role as their supervisor. As a registrar, you accept that your role requires your participation in the on-call roster. Roles are usually complementary. For example, for you to take the role of doctor, someone else must agree to take the role of patient. To be in the role of teacher, someone else must be willing to be in the role of student.

You may have experienced a situation where roles are not clear or not agreed by the actors, this is not a sustainable position and can involve a lot of conflict, resistance, time, and energy. Role clarity is important in effective teamwork and can affect your sense of self in terms of safety, performance, and wellbeing. Like all the work we are doing in this book, it is helpful to get clear on your role and the expectations that come with it.

Your role at work is potentially an expression of your self, though not necessarily. Your self is not the same as your role:

- Does *doctor* describe the whole of you or only part of you?
- What other words would you use to describe your role at work as a doctor?

Here are a few options that doctors have suggested to me over the years to describe their role: healer, scientist, fixer, facilitator, expert.

- Do any of these resonate with you?
- How do you respond to each of these descriptions of your doctor role?

> **Your self is the sum of your experiences, energy, values and beliefs – as determined by you.**

Your *self* is determined by you and is the essence of you, determined by what *you* relate to, what you do, and how you show up in the world. The work here is to know your self rather than limit your personal development to the roles you play.

Your self-determined *self* is what makes you a unique individual. The story you tell yourself about whether you are funny or brave or capable comes from your internal world as you have distilled your experience. You take something from every role you have inhibited into your self, what you notice is unique to you. Your perception and interpretation are based on what you believe and value and where you place your attention and awareness.

> Your self and your role as doctor overlap or even conflate. You might even lose your sense of self in your role.

## Self - Role

Completely
Overlap

Dynamic

Authenticity

Role                Self

Completely
Separate

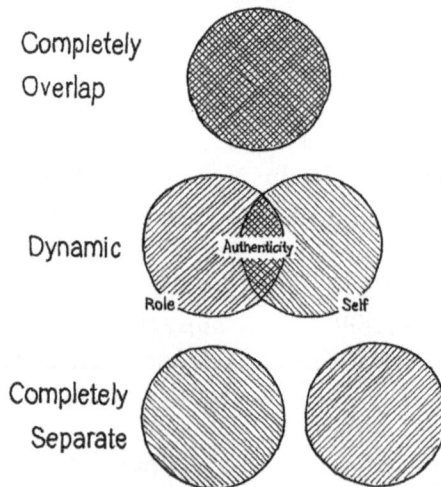

This image demonstrates the dynamic nature of self and role. Your work environment ascribes expectations and assumptions to you in your role of doctor. You bring your sense of self either consciously or unconsciously. You might experience total overlap of role and self as in the first image. Or a total disconnect as in the third image. Both positions have their inherent risks and potential benefits.

The strategy of complete separation of self and role has worked for some, but for many the energy it takes to maintain this separation is tiring. Some doctors understand being professional as leaving their emotions at the door – this is a version of self and role separation. A separation some doctors describe as soul destroying and others claim as their sanity. A doctor who brings little of their self to their role can seem mysterious, aloof, or disconnected to their colleagues and patients and never seem fully present. As a result, levels of trust and psychological safety can remain low. Humans connect with each other via their emotions as much as their thinking.

Equally, if your role and self are totally in sync (as in the top image), you might experience a loss of self. To give you an example, a doctor who is retiring after working 70 hours a week for 40 years in one hospital, might find it difficult to envisage themself separate from their role, and their retirement could create an extreme identity crisis. I remember one military doctor who was being discharged telling me he didn't know who he was without his uniform.

The separated position (on the right) is usually a protective position. If you are coming to work as a doctor like this, it is likely that you are concerned in some way about your psychological safety. This position is not usually sustainable for long. Even a small amount of overlap is more sustainable, giving you a sense of authenticity as you align some of your values and meaning with your role. Feeling even some small level of personal connection to the role, the work, the team or the patients is more sustainable. I encourage you to find some values-based connection to your work beyond your role, no matter how slim the overlap, it will make your work more meaningful and more sustainable.

## Brendon's Story

*Brendon, a consultant, described to me the revelation he had after presenting some of his research to the medical directors of various departments in his hospital. The presentation was in-person and it was important to him, as it represented a potential breakthrough in the way patients in his speciality would be treated. Brendon is one of only a handful of people who have the skills and knowledge in his area. As an expert walking a fine line – convincing his seniors to look at integrating what he was finding into their patient-facing work without sounding evangelistic – he had felt anxious.*

*He told me he was pleased with his presentation and that it had been well received. The big surprise was that the medical director of the hospital had been present, but Brendon hadn't realised because some people were there via phone and zoom. He said if he had known the chief medical director was present, he would not have presented in the same way – he would have been more nervous and would have tried to sound "more professorial". As it was, the CMD was delighted with the presentation and phoned him to say so.*

*Brendon learnt that he could be authentic in the way he spoke, that he did not need to change the way he spoke for people to resonate with his work and the way he discussed it. He learnt that he could safely bring more of his self to his role than he had predicted, and that it felt great. Coaching raised his awareness and commitment to bringing more of his self to work. Brendon said it felt better on this occasion, but it also made him feel nervous and he thought it likely that he would unconsciously revert to his habit of trying to look and sound more professorial than he felt. The work continues for Brendon as he consciously chooses authenticity.*

Doctors often express their worry to me about their presence and how they are perceived by their colleagues. Some are concerned about appearing too arrogant or confident, and others worry that they do not present as confident enough. Only you can work out the right balance. Both an inflated ego and a deflated ego can be problematic in terms of balancing self and role. Your ego is engaged in protecting your *self* and is focused on making sure you are valued, recognised and ideally praised. As you grow your self-awareness you will become more skilled in understanding how to wisely work with your ego and your inner critic. In the first instance, remember that self and role are highly dynamic, and the expression of your *self* is highly dependent on your psychological safety.

The overlap between your role and self is your authentic self

– finding the right amount of authenticity is contextual, organic and highly dynamic. As with everything I have discussed in Chapters 3 and 4, the more aware you are of your internal environment, the better you can regulate yourself, meeting your own needs and consequently those of the people you serve more effectively. It helps you bring enough of your true self to your role of doctor. Reflecting with someone you trust like a coach is a robust and expansive process that supports this kind of development.

> When you have done this internal work of regulation and deep knowing, the roles you take and how you deliver them are likely to change.

## SUMMARY

Medical training is competency based, little time or energy is spent understanding the *person* who is training to become a doctor.

> Ignoring the person who is the doctor is a self-limiting strategy, your human desires and aversions are activating your behaviour all the time, including at work.

Figuring out who you are is a lifelong project. Developing a sense of self includes establishing your values and forming your own distinct identity – separating yourself from your parents, and continuing to clarify what you want for yourself, as opposed to what others say you should do and be.

Knowing your beliefs, values and purpose creates an internal foundation you can rely upon. Listen to your own voice with mindfulness and self-compassion.

> Embracing this work creates intimate knowledge of your inner world and facilitates agency, helping you do more and be more of what you love.

When you have a warm relationship with yourself, deeply attuned to your own needs, desires, aversions and meaning making, your influence and relationships with others change in positive ways, sometimes incrementally and sometimes as transformation, both are useful. In this way, meaning making facilitates the other four elements of PERMA - positive emotions, more engagement, effective relationships, and achievement, helping you to do more than survive medicine – helping you flourish.

### Actions for knowing yourself

1. Understand what you seek so you can focus your effort meaningfully, this is your purpose anchor.
2. Unearth and name your primary beliefs – decide which ones serve you well. Consider letting some go.
3. Identify your core values. Along with your purpose anchors, these are your guides.
4. Make values-based decisions, reduce the amount of cognitive dissonance you hold.
5. Create an external scaffold of habits and trusted people to help you deliver committed actions aligned with your values and purpose.
6. Practise! Skills come first. Confidence grows as a result of skill.
7. Practise recognising your role as distinct from your self. Notice the dynamic nature of their overlap. Make sure there is enough of an overlap to feel authentic in your role.

# 5 | RELIEVE STRESS

## Naomi's Story

*Naomi worked as an advanced trainee obstetrician and gynaecologist. She moved hospitals every six months as part of her training program, including to regional areas. For weeks at a time, she was away from her partner and young children, focusing on her goal to fellow. I met her when she had just arrived at a regional city rotation and was studying for her exam, which was three months away.*

*During her last shift at her 'parent' hospital in the city, her supervisor had given her the collective feedback from the consultants she had been working with. Most of it was great, but someone had said she needed to work on her confidence, that she wasn't yet behaving like a consultant.*

*Moving to a new hospital with no familiar colleagues, no knowledge of the region or the hospital processes, and no support network was stressful. In her new rotation, Naomi felt anxious. The feedback had confused her and was playing on her mind. It was vague and behavioural examples had not been provided.*

*She began the rotation on nights by herself. Within a couple of hours of one shift, there were three women giving birth, two with complications, and one of those with twins. She had not met any of the consultants working at the new hospital, but on this night she definitely needed to call someone. Yet now she was overthinking what it would look like if she was seen to be asking for help so early.*

*When we met a few days later, Naomi was wracked with doubt and anxiety, and was extremely tired. She said, "If I don't pass this exam, I don't know what I'm going to do." She was totally unsupported at her regional hospital. Her role as trainee was swamping the rest of her life, her self. She needed to learn to separate what was a stressor in her environment from the internal stress response she was feeling. Only then could she begin improving her own situation.*

## DISTINGUISH STRESS FROM STRESSORS

Being a doctor involves a lot of stress. Distinguishing stressors from the stress response in your body will help you respond much more effectively than using the general idea of being stressed. For Naomi, identifying the vague consultant feedback as a stressor helped direct our work in coaching. So did recognising that the stressors at the new hospital changed rapidly as she got to know people and processes. Naming the specific factors that were causing stress made a big difference to her stress level.

In this chapter, we will review how you can understand the stress response and its opposite, the relaxation response, for your benefit. We will take a closer look at how your improving self-awareness and the skills of self-regulation and can set you up to manage stress better.

> **Knowing about the physiology of stress doesn't always mean you are good at managing stress in your own life.**

## YOUR STRESSORS ARE YOURS TO MANAGE

Managing stress effectively means being able to identify the factors in your life that make you feel stressed - the **stressors**. Which factors create stress for you is unique and personal. The same factor may not trigger the person next to you. Talking about stress in general terms isn't especially helpful in regards to knowing how to respond.

For example, I find it incredibly stressful if a cat walks past me and rubs against my legs. Many people find it ridiculous that I am triggered by a small friendly animal! The cat is a stressor in my environment for me personally. It is not a stressor for most other people. If a cat comes along, I *feel* stressed. My mind starts telling me stories of being scratched and triggers my body's stress response. It doesn't matter what other's think, it doesn't even matter what my own rational mind thinks, I am still stressed when a cat is around.

The cat itself is not stress, the cat is triggering *my* stress response, changing my internal environment because of what I believe and pay attention to. *My* stress response is caused by *my* thoughts about the cat, which in this case come from my history. For others, a cat will trigger their relaxation response, the opposite physiological reaction to the stress response. For many, a cat won't trigger any change of state at all. Naming the stressor gives me a focus for action, it allows me to be responsive instead of reactive.

How you respond to life, what you think about it, affects your performance and your wellbeing. These factors are intimately interconnected. You can leverage your performance and your wellbeing up or down by the way you think about the stressors in your life. These thinking patterns are not always conscious though; they can be triggered by your brain well before you have any awareness of what's happening. Your thinking can also be distorted if you are depleted (remember HALLTSS from Chapter 3) so there is a limit to how many stressors you can pile on.

Naming the stressors helps you take specific action to remove or attend to them. Managing the stressors that remain requires your skilful internal response.

> Naming your stressors allows you to respond more effectively, creating opportunities to leverage and influence your performance and your wellbeing, improving your sense of balance and your opportunity to thrive.

## STRESS IS NOT NECESSARILY BAD

Stress itself is not bad, in fact it's incredibly useful in the right dose. Another way to think about stress is to think of being *activated*.

When world champion surfer Mick Fanning was filmed fighting off a shark in 2015 in the J-Bay Open World Surfing League in South Africa, you could see that his body was fully activated. Before he consciously processed the shark was there, his brain had already triggered his stress response: more blood was directed to his muscles, his mind became single focused, his heart and lungs were working at maximum capacity, his digestive and reproductive systems shut down and his sight and hearing were automatically turned up.

Mick's body would have been activated at a low level already, he was after all surfing in an international competition. But as a seasoned world champion, he may not have been *aware* of much activation.

When the shark took a swipe at Mick's board, his body amped up the level of stress response activation in a millisecond. The shark was a much more threatening stressor than any surfing competition could be for him at that moment. His automatic responses kept him alive much more effectively than his slow conscious prefrontal cortex processes could have.

This activation happened quickly, automatically and powerfully to meet the high-level threat to his survival. A minute later, safely on a rescue boat, Mick was shaking from the adrenaline surge. This kind of threat to survival activates humans instantly, and then takes just minutes to a few hours for our physiologically to return to baseline.

How often is your body activating as if there is a shark in the water? If your body is maintaining your stress response continuously, it will be difficult for you to achieve a sense of balance and it is unlikely that you will have the necessary energy for agency in your own life. This is an unsustainable position and puts you and your patients at risk. Chronic activation of the stress response dysregulates you and clear thinking becomes near impossible.

Most of us, most of the time, can successfully integrate the stressful experiences of our lives with the right tools and the right support. Thankfully, Mick survived and has become an advocate for sharks, demonstrating clearly how a person with the right tools and support can take a highly stressful event and integrate it into their life. He serves as a clear example of how the feeling of being stressed can evolve differently: it can resolve and be integrated into our lives, or it can continue on as a chronic problem. The stressor is only an ongoing problem because of the story you tell yourself, not because it exists.

> Your internal environment – what you believe, value, pay attention to, are aware of – affects how much stress you experience.

Whether something triggers your stress response or not can change over time, it's contextual. The very same trigger can be stressful sometimes and not be other times, for the same person.

## YOUR BODY ONLY HAS ONE PHYSIOLOGICAL RESPONSE TO STRESSORS

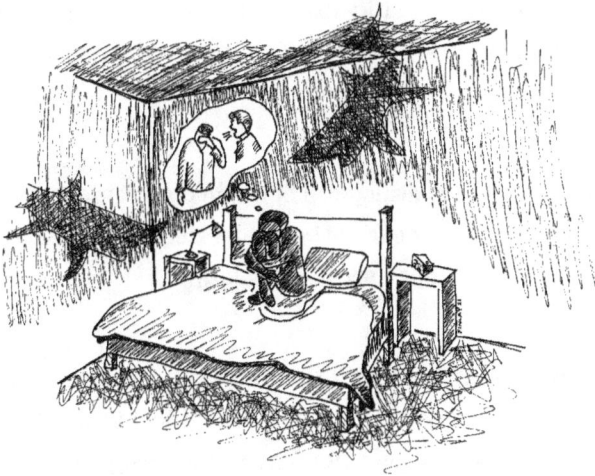

Your body only has one stress response – the same cascade of neurochemicals, hormones and other physiological changes happens in all situations that are stressful for you. If you are lying in your bed and dream of a shark attacking you, your body will activate in the same way as if it's really happening. If you are at work and feel like the supervisor or consultant is going to challenge or embarrass you, your body will react the same way. If you are asked to perform a procedure you have never done before, that can be terrifying and will activate the same physiological stress response.

> Your physiological responses to stress are the same whether you imagine, anticipate, remember, or are actually in the middle of a terrifying event.

Once you identify the stressors in your life, you can do something about them. Being specific about your stressors is important. Saying you are stressed in a generalised way does not show you what you can do to improve the situation. Victor Frankl managed his stress in Auschwitz concentration camp by focusing his attention on his hope of meeting his wife again one day. Mick Fanning managed his post shark attack stress by learning as much as he could about sharks.

Can you name the specific stressors in your life that are triggering your stress response? Be as specific as possible. How do you want to respond to them? You get to choose.

> The first step is to distinguish between the stressors in your life and your experience of being stressed. Identify what is uniquely stressful for you.

Perhaps you are stressed by the number of patients you need to see in clinic, or a particular consultant whom you feel intimidated by, or the nurse unit manager who shows her frustration easily when you are indecisive, or the idea of deciding what you will eat for dinner after a 12 hour shift, or the interview process you need to go through to keep your job for another year, or inserting a canula into a young child. Perhaps you are stressed about how you misdiagnosed a patient because you were stressed in the ED or so overwhelmed by how many patients were waiting for you.

> There are thousands of potential stressors in your life. Practise naming them specifically.

## PERCEIVING STRESS – THE STORY YOU TELL YOURSELF

The wrong response to stress can be fatal. In fact, researchers have found that our *beliefs* about stress might be more important than the stressor in terms of our wellbeing. Keller, Litzelman, Wisket et al (2012) looked at a representative sample of people in the US between 1998 and 2006. They looked at the national health interview survey and the national death index to understand the impact of the amount of stress in a person's life, their perception of how stress affected their health, and who died prematurely.

They found that a high amount of stress plus a perception that stress affects health negatively, increased a person's risk of premature death by 43%. Importantly, they also found that people who had lots of stress in their life but did not regard it as harmful, were no more likely to die prematurely than people with the lowest levels of stress in their lives. The people with high stress but no negative perceptions about it had the lowest risk of dying prematurely.

> The biggest risk factor for dying prematurely from stress related causes is having the perception that stress is bad for you.

## ACTIVITY 8

**Try this:**

1.  Learn to recognise your specific stressors. Notice and name them.

2.  Practise labelling your body's stress response as **activation**. Words are important –what happens when you say to yourself "I'm activated" instead of saying "I'm stressed"?

Do you feel or think differently?

Are you more aware of a sense of choice and agency, rather than feeling like a victim or being trapped?

3.  Try it out for the next week, each time you notice a story you are telling yourself about stress, replace the word *stressed* with *activated*. Be curious, pay attention, and see what you learn.

## FIND YOUR ACTIVATION SWEET SPOT

Yerkes and Dodson first described the stress curve in 1908 to explain the relationship between pressure and performance, demonstrating that arousal increases performance but only up to a point, and then performance decreases. When it comes to your body being aroused, it is not the case that more is better. Too much stress causes your internal system to be overwhelmed. Not enough stress will make it hard for you to generate energy and focus. The sweet spot is enough stress – activation – to achieve your goals.

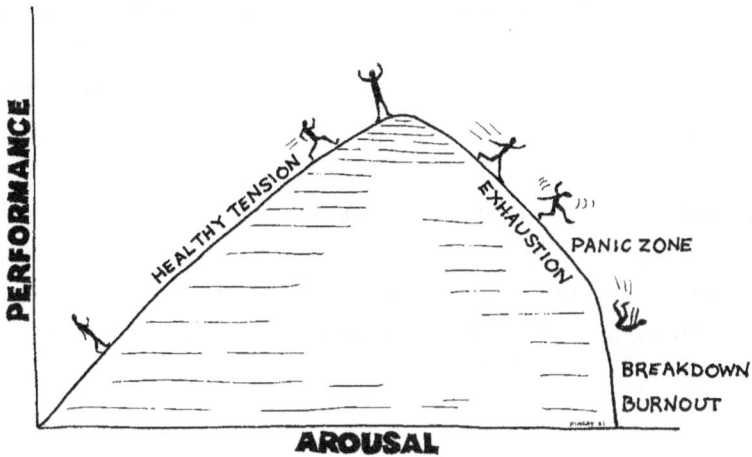

Where you are on the stress curve will differ depending on your activity. If you are doing a difficult or novel task, you will not need as much activation (stress) to perform as well as when you are doing something that requires persistence or stamina.

As a trainee surgeon, for example, you will not need much activation to help you focus and concentrate on learning a new surgical technique, you will be naturally present because the activity is novel and perhaps the risk to patient safety is high. If you are also feeling intimidated by your supervisor and this is triggering your stress response as well, you could easily be over aroused and feel overwhelmed, pushing you over the top of the stress curve, reducing your performance. You might describe this as being too stressed.

In activities that are routine or require long-term concentration or commitment, you will need to be more aroused for peak performance to keep you motivated. Your experience of stress depends on:

- the activity itself
- the environment
- your internal response (your perception/story).

Your body is aroused (or not) by the environment and by your perception of whether you have the resources required to meet the need or not. You can actively and intentionally change your stress experience. People describe feeling stressed at all points on the Yerkes-Dodson curve. In fact, people in the lower reaches of the curve, to the left where there is low activation or arousal, often feel high levels of stress – like an experienced general surgeon who is bored by years of endoscopes. They could raise their activation by taking on a registrar and teaching them, making endoscopes more interesting or challenging and pushing them further up the curve. By changing the circumstances and the way you respond to them, you create more internal activation for yourself.

## A SENSE OF CONTROL REDUCES YOUR FEELING OF STRESS

One way to reduce your experience of stress is to increase your sense of control over the work you do. Leaders often experience less stress even though they have more responsibility, because they have more of a sense of control over their activities. A junior doctor has less ability to control their environment which can activate the stress response and keep it activated. Perception is important – choose your focus.

Ritual and routine can help you feel a sense of control. One doctor told me if they could park their car in their preferred spot, they achieved a sense of control. Another doctor described knowing their roster three months in advance had given them this sense of control in their broader life, and it was enough to then tolerate the chaos when they were at work. These doctors were choosing their focus, which helped them feel less stressed.

Finding ways to control even small parts of your work, perceiving your own autonomy and agency where you can and looking for ways to be authentic to your own values can reduce your feeling of being stressed.

In the right amount, stress helps you focus, activate, and achieve. High achievers and top performers know how to work effectively with stress. They operate in the top of the Yerkes-Dodson's stress curve for optimum performance.

They are aware of:

- where they are in terms of arousal and performance
- adjusting the environment to reduce or raise their level of challenge
- the value of rest and recovery
- their responsibility to take action when they need a break.

Deciding to take a break is another way to induce a small sense of control in your life.

Even in horrible situations, you can use your agency to stabilise yourself. The thriving doctor will focus on meaning, achievement, the relationships involved, and their ability to engage. They will practise gratitude for what is working, generating positive emotion out of the other PERMA elements.

> **Thriving doctors are not without stress, they simply know how to use it to their advantage.**

They understand that more stress does not equal more productivity or more effectiveness. They think systemically and recognise the balancing properties of rest, recovery, and boundaries. They notice that too much activation (stress) can overwhelm them and lead to apathy, hopelessness, reduced performance and illness. They have learnt by paying attention and cultivating awareness over time, how much activation is too much for them. When this is aligned with their beliefs and their values, they are able to manage more of what they activate towards and when they need to create a boundary.

## BALANCING THE STRESS RESPONSE AND THE RELAXATION RESPONSE

You can think of your body when it has activated your stress response as going into the red zone (sympathetic dominance). You might also describe it as being in a state of fight or flight. The opposite state is the relaxation response. This is the state the human body is designed to be in the majority of the time. Your parasympathetic nervous system is more active in this state (sometimes called rest and digest). You can think of your body's relaxation response as the green zone.

### *The Red Zone*

Let's refresh your biology briefly. An important part of survival is keeping your body in balance, homeostasis. When your brain perceives a threat, your amygdala sounds the alarm, instantly activating a cascade of physiological changes. Your blood stream is awash with neurochemicals, principally cortisol, adrenaline, noradrenaline, and testosterone. Your sympathetic nervous system is dominating all your systems and overriding your prefrontal cortex, making rational thinking less available, limiting reflective thinking, and reducing your ability to relate to others effectively. This leaves you feeling agitated, disengaged, or wanting to avoid the situation all together. You are on high alert, ready to fight or run in a desperate attempt to maintain or regain control.

While you are in the red zone, you have less access to hormones like oxytocin which helps you bond and attach to others, serotonin which helps you feel calm, and melatonin which initiates the sleep cycle every 24 hours. If you stay in the red zone, cortisol and adrenaline build up, degrading tissue, undermining your immune system, disrupting your digestion, reproduction and cardiovascular health, and interfering with your sleep, which in turn causes headaches, high blood pressure, sexual dysfunction, and hypervigilance. Over the long term, living in the red zone cultivates the conditions for depression and anxiety, psychological distress, disease and, worst of all, suicide.

Is this how you live? Many doctors describe this state to me as their "normal". If you live in the red zone most of the time, it's going to be difficult to achieve balance. To create something different in your life will mean changing. It will help to have some supporters around you. Sometimes the first skill you need to develop is sharing your experience with someone who cares about you. Tell someone you trust about what you are working on and choose one small change to commit to. Perhaps it's going to bed 15 minutes earlier or deciding to say no to a recent invitation to a meeting that is not critical to your work and does not give you joy.

Your brain and body systems in the red zone are extremely efficient. Unfortunately that can sometimes lead us awry. Your systems use short fast assessments like good/bad and right/wrong. You are much more prone to bias, and your thinking is cognitively rigid as you revert to old established patterns and your existing cognitive templates. The higher order thinking of your pre-frontal cortex goes offline.

This is why training for emergencies with checklists, easily remembered mnemonics, and agreed protocols, is critical. It's all about efficiency in the red zone. You are effectively tapping into what your body does naturally in an emergency, using instinct and following patterns that have been embedded over and over through practice. Emergency services, the military, aviation, and medicine alike train these patterns into their people for time limited situations like when CPR is required. Your body is designed to react quickly and effectively in the red zone as a spike, not as a permanently elevated flatline.

## The Green Zone

The relaxation response is the green zone. It is the opposite body state to the red zone. Your body is exquisitely designed to exist in the relaxation response most of the time. It's where you can learn, feed and reproduce. Our thinking in the green zone is controlled by our pre-frontal cortex and is more reflective. We are able to challenge, correct, be creative, generate new ideas and see new links. In the relaxed state, you are perceptive and flexible because you think and feel psychologically safe. You are more capable of human connection and more aware of our interdependence when you are in the green zone state. It's all about effectiveness in the green zone.

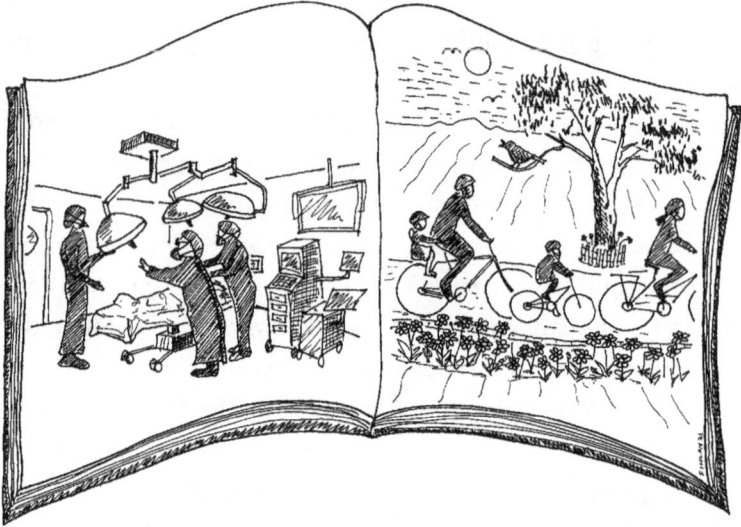

For hundreds of thousands of years, people have lived in the green zone with only occasional sharp peaks of activation into the red zone state in response to threat. Now, too many doctors live in the red zone too much of the time, making them cognitively rigid, blaming the system and having no idea how to change the situation. It doesn't have to be this way.

You can raise your awareness and learn how to live more in the green zone *even though* you work in medicine. Start with one simple step and build from there. Start by naming your stressors, when you can notice what they are. Start observing if you are in the red or the green zone.

> Stress helps you achieve your goals. Learning how to harness the energy of your activated body might be the difference between your success and failure in medicine.

Be your own agent of change to manage the stressors in your life. Making any change requires that you notice that there is some behaviour or activity that is no longer serving you. Perhaps in naming the stressors in your life, noticing your red zone triggers, you have observed something you need to change in your life. Once you have noticed what needs changing, you need to be able to describe it accurately. The work you have done in Chapters 3 and 4 has probably helped you name what is important to you and may have also pointed toward some of the key stressors in your life. When you can name the stressor, you can start to tame it.

> The umbrella term 'stress' is too general. Name your specific stressors that put you into the red zone. Now you can respond to them more usefully.

You can learn to move out of the red zone towards the green zone and stabilise yourself. Mindfulness cultivates the awareness you need to notice which zone you are operating in, and to course correct for well-being and better performance. By consciously regulating, rather than defaulting unconsciously out of habit to a reactive red zone state, you can take better care of yourself and your patients.

In the example below, each of these steps is underlined to help you see the process in action.

*Imagine you are working in the emergency department. It's 11pm on a Saturday night. It's the middle of winter and two doctors have called in sick. Everything seems too slow; patients are waiting too long, pathology is slow, the beds are full, ambulances are ramping, the triage nurse is agitated, someone in the waiting room has just started to scream. You haven't had anything to eat or drink since you started four hours ago. Your stress response is activated, whether you notice it in the moment or not. You are getting deeper and deeper into the red zone.*

*As you move between the patients and consulting with your colleagues, you notice that your energy is dipping. You go over to the water filter, pausing to take a couple of mouthfuls of water. Your mind is full of thoughts about how you can possibly keep up with two doctors down. You worry about making a mistake and feel frustrated about the pathology results you're waiting on. You notice that you are feeling a bit anxious, you name the feeling to yourself ("anxiety is here"). As you do, you remember that your intention as you arrived at work today was to practise raising your awareness. You label your experience again to yourself, saying, "anxiety is here and my stress response is activated." Just noticing and saying this is validating and seems to help you process the emotions. You feel a little steadier.*

*You choose to take one long, slow breath out to help reengage your pre-frontal cortex and balance your nervous system. This helps you let go of the critical and blaming judgements that were gathering in your mind, creating tension in your body. You are more present to your own body now, so you drink a little more water. You make your way to the next patient feeling stabilised. As you walk, you focus on your feet feeling the floor, this simple mindful practice is grounding and brings you into the present moment. You arrive at the next patient's bed feeling steady, focused, and clear of mind having interrupted the slide into deep red zone territory.*

## YOUR INNER VOICE:
## THE STORY YOU TELL YOURSELF IS A STRESSOR TOO

The external environment has the potential to sling arrows (stressors) at you all day and night: demanding patients, rude consultants, energy-sucking colleagues, daunting college processes, complicated funding agreements, your family and friends needing more of you, governments who fail to provide information and resources, inflammatory media. The list of ways in which the environment can stress you out is only limited by your imagination. These external stressors are the first arrows.

Your response to these realities – your thoughts about them – are like a second round of arrows that you shoot at yourself. These are your perceptions of stress in your life, the story you tell yourself. Remember Keller et al's study which found that people who died prematurely often were the people who *thought* that stress was bad for them. These people were creating a second round of arrows to sling at themselves. Psychologists call these *amplifiers*. You might have experienced them in the dead of night or when you have been isolated from your community and family. Thought patterns like rumination and catastrophising are examples of second arrows, amplifiers.

Second arrow thoughts might sound like this: "I don't think I am up to this, I don't have enough skill, I'm not experienced enough, I should have seen that coming, other people seem to be able to manage their finances better than me, I need to manage my time more effectively, someone will soon discover what an imposter I am, I'm scared of that consultant, if I don't get onto the training program I won't have a job or any kind of future." Second arrows are generated by your thinking and are felt as fear, anxiety and distress.

> You cannot change most of the first-round arrows, the stressors that the world throws at you. You can use your values and the self-regulation skills you are practising so you do not create so many second arrows. You can manage your internal response and stop amplifying the stressors in your life.

Here's an example of the double arrows concept to help bring this to life for you. Remember when you were studying for a difficult, important exam. The reality of your life then might have included exam related first arrows that looked something like this:

- Complex content including Latin names and precise details to remember
- Limited support, living away from home, isolated from friends and family
- Lack of time – cook, clean, buy groceries for self
- No social fun in life for a long time, no easy way to relax
- Exhausted – working full time and studying when tired
- Hospital colleagues who were rude, impatient, demanding
- Knowing that only 50% of people the year before passed this exam.

Possible second arrows might have included thoughts or ruminations like these:

- I will never remember all of this, I'm too tired and not smart enough.
- I was crazy to think I could manage this, I miss my mum, what a baby I am.
- I hate cooking dinner, I'm getting Macca's again, it's pathetic, I'm embarrassed by the way I eat, I know it's bad, I'm a doctor for goodness' sake!
- All I want to do is sleep, I should be able to get it together, what's wrong with me?
- I know I'm going to fail, what's the point of even trying?
- Who do I think I am? I should give up. How can my family have sacrificed so much for me?

## ACTIVITY 9

### Raise your awareness to second arrows

You can start expanding your self-awareness by reflecting on the previous example and answering the following 7 questions.

1. What did you do, or not do, so that you could pass your last exam?

2. How did you meet the demands of the external environment? What did you do that was actually useful?

3. How did you respond to your internal environment? What did you do that was actually useful?

4. What skills do you notice now on reflection that you need in order to be more effective going forward?

5. What values did you anchor yourself with?

6. What are you now aware of?

7. How can you cultivate more of this awareness?

You can use these questions to raise your awareness about how you are responding to any first arrow.

## PAIN IS A GIVEN, SUFFERING IS OPTIONAL

The problem or pain is the first arrow. These are largely unavoidable in life. COVID-19 is a first arrow, and how you think about it could be a second arrow. Second arrows amplify the impact of the first arrow, creating suffering. Suffering is optional. Let me walk you through an equation that might help you look at the role you play in turning pain into suffering. Please replace the word pain with problem if that makes more sense to you.

It is human to initially resist when something goes wrong that causes you pain as part of orienting to a new situation and planning your response. Imagine your car breaks down and you have to wait for someone to help you, which makes you late. This causes you pain; it's natural to feel annoyed. If you are in a useful state of mind, you will soon shift your focus and set about resolving the situation.

When something unexpected and unwanted goes wrong, it is normal to express your emotions, complain, fret, ruminate and catastrophise. Doing this for a short while might even help you feel better, especially if you do it out loud by talking to someone you trust, and they do it too. This process is better thought of as co-brooding and has the benefit of creating bonds in trusting relationships. For the most part however, people who complain are miserable. This complaining, ruminating, and ongoing grumbling can be described as resistance.

Pain is amplified by resistance, which turns it into suffering. People who can move more readily to problem solving, action or acceptance experience less suffering. They still have problems and pain in their lives, but they are not exacerbating the experience in a negative direction. They are not labouring under a round of second arrows.

The next time you are thinking about a problem in your life, apply this equation and see if it helps you to defuse your thinking and in turn reduce or detach a little from your internal resistance. Then observe how you relate to your problem or your pain. You might like to think about the first and second arrows using this equation:

$$\text{Pain x Resistance} = \text{Suffering}$$
$$10 \text{ x } 10 = 100$$
$$10 \text{ x } 0 = 0 \text{ Suffering}$$

Let me show you how you can use this equation.

*Imagine you had an adverse event at work – someone died and now there is a coroner's inquiry into what happened. You were the decision maker in the situation. The pain is as high as it can be for you, give it 10 units. You go home feeling completely desolate and numb. Your colleagues have been encouraging, saying that no one could have anticipated the series of events as they happened. The medical director came to see you before you left work and explained the process, saying he'd talk with you again tomorrow, that you should come to work as normal. He was warm and encouraging, doing his best to support you.*

*Now you are at home crying, but you can't bring yourself to tell your family what has happened. Eventually, in the middle of the night, you tell your partner because you can't sleep. Your body activated the stress response hours ago before the patient died. It has stayed on high alert – as it is designed to do under such serious threat conditions – despite the fact that there is no actual immediate threat.*

*Your mind is going over and over what happened. Other than the patient notes at work, you haven't written anything down out of fear of someone reading it and your being found to have got it wrong. It's hard to remember the exact series of events or the exact words you used anyway. Your mind is telling you all sorts of hypervigilant contradictory stories, like:* I'm going to lose my job, my colleagues must hate me, the other consultant said they would have done the same – were they just being kind? The family will never ever forgive me, I should have been an electrician, next time I meet a patient like this I'm going to freeze up, I need to move interstate, I'm so ashamed, the consultant said I did the right thing but they weren't there... I bet they would have got it right. *You are suffering enormously.*

Most of these thoughts are resistance – second arrows. Your resistance is at 10 too, amplifying the pain. They arise for good reason; your brain is trying to predict what will happen next so it can protect you. Your ego might also get involved, looking to blame others or thinking about escape routes as protection mechanisms. None of this is wrong, but all of it amplifies the pain causing you to suffer.

A person who is highly skilled in mindfulness, self-compassion and emotional intelligence has the skills to manage this pain more effectively, responding to the pain that exists without so much amplifying. If we use the equation above, they might experience three or four units of resistance rather than 10. As a compassionate and connected person, any adverse event will be challenging in your role as a doctor. When things go wrong, you are reminded that you are a fallible human and because of that it is natural to suffer. With the right skills and the right support around you, your response to pain can be more effective, meaning that you use your energy, effort and time more usefully, responding to the pain without amplifying it. You can hold your balance, maintaining clarity and personal agency.

Experiment with this equation as part of your response to whatever stressors you currently have in your life. Perhaps it is even useful to help you think through some problem you currently have. Writing in your journal or talking a problem through with someone you trust can help you identify your resistance. These are factors we can control, they are largely thoughts, so once you have identified them you have the opportunity to respond differently.

In this example, you might even amplify the advice and encouragement you received from your colleagues and the medical director, sharing that with your partner. Perhaps you can say the coroner is investigating because it is unclear and has not happened before, rather than jumping to the conclusion that it was your fault. This reframing process is about gaining perspective rather than getting sucked into a vortex of suffering. Remembering the Just-World Hypothesis might also help – the world is not just or fair, luck plays a role, bad things happening are not caused because you are 'bad', the world is unpredictable with many uncontrollable factors at play.

> Your beliefs and stories about stress are more harmful than the stress
> itself. Most stressors will not kill you, but your reaction to them might.
> Stress does not have to become suffering.

## YOUR PSYCHOLOGICAL NEEDS

The three basic psychological needs of an adult are to be safe (survive), to belong, and to achieve (sometimes called autonomy). When we feel unsafe, isolated, and unable to progress, we are at great risk. When we feel safe, like we belong, and that we have the opportunity and resources to set our own course, we can meet an impressive number of stressors in our life.

### Reflection

- Do you feel safe at work in your role?
- What factors contribute to you feeling safe or not?
- Do you feel a sense of belonging in the medical community? At your workplace?
- Are you able to do work that gives you a sense of autonomy?
- Do you feel like you are achieving something meaningful in your work?

When things are stressful and demand is greater than your resources, you need other people. That is part of the human condition. While we can manage on our own for a while, there are no exceptions in the long term. Humans have a deeply rooted need to feel connected. You were a person well before you became a doctor. You can ameliorate your stress by building a community, or several communities, that you feel connected to. I encourage you to build meaningful connections in your medical communities and outside of medicine so that you are taking care of your self, not just in your role as doctor. Remember PERMA includes feeling engaged, positive relationships, meaning and a sense of achievement.

> The more psychologically safe you feel, the more trust you have in the group. The more able to make mistakes you are, the more you can learn and grow.

When it comes to autonomy (achievement) what gives you the most satisfaction? Are you giving that activity your best energy and effort? Have you ever had a hobby or a cause that you have happily given your free time to? Stayed up late in the night to fit it in around your other commitments just because you can, and you want to? Ever been involved in something at work that doesn't feel like work? You might have heard yourself say, "I'd do it for free, I don't really care if they pay me". These are examples of autonomy – you are choosing to do it simply because you can. You are involved because you want to be. Achieving in this environment is easy, stress or activation feels natural, you don't ponder about energy, effort or even time. When this opportunity to choose is limited, adults push back.

We have seen this in the pandemic. Lockdowns have restricted our movements even within our own neighbourhoods. Even though they might not have wanted to go anywhere, the fact that someone else had imposed a rule made many adults feel upset, their choice was taken away. This is my preferred word for the psychological need for autonomy or achievement – choice. Adults want to feel their own agency in their life. They want to be able to 'do it their way'.

Many primary care doctors who used to work in smaller clinics and now work in super clinics or corporate clinics describe losing their sense of independence and autonomy. Do you ever feel more like a resource than an independent thinking expert? This change in perceived status and control is a contributor to stress. Most of the patients and their ailments remain the same, the work looks the same, but the doctor's experience is different. In this scenario, your sense of autonomy and independence has changed, you may not feel like you are able to make your own choices and this shift can lead to feeling more stressed. There are some different stressors in the system and your relationship to your work may have changed.

Remember Shanafelt et al's research which found that doctors need to be able to choose 20% of their work activities to prevent burnout. This choice is meeting the need for autonomy.

It is also a form of achievement when you meet your own psychological needs, as this evokes positive emotion, meaning you feel better resourced and more able to meet the needs of your environment and the demands of your life. The stressors might be the same, but you are different. You are more capable, more effective, and more sustainable.


## HOW TO TAKE CARE OF YOURSELF: THE STORY YOU TELL YOURSELF

Remember when you inserted your first catheter or canula while your supervisor or the NUM was watching? Whether you were fearful and anxious, or excited and motivated, your stress response was activated and your body released adrenaline. If you were anxious, you might have felt upset, tried to avoid doing it, or felt ashamed or embarrassed. If you were excited, you might have felt focused and energised. If you were anxious, you might have had thoughts like *what if I mess it up or hurt the patient or have to ask for help, I feel sick, if I faint or cry I will be so embarrassed.* If you were excited, you might have had thoughts like *now I really feel like I can be a doctor, I'm looking forward to contributing to looking after this person, it's exciting to actually practise my new skills.* Your stress response was triggered, your mind created a story to explain what was happening and your emotions arose as a result of the way your mind predicted the outcomes. Then your mind created some more stories to describe what was happening. This cycle is happening constantly.

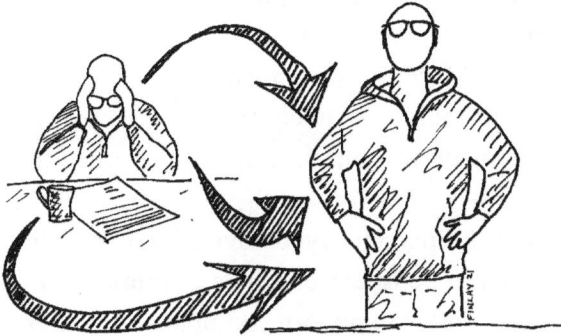

Whether you experience anxiety or excitement, the stress response is activating you. Once you become consciously aware of what's happening, you create an opportunity to choose how you respond. If you have done the work of earlier chapters and you are clear about your values, then you can use them as anchors to orient yourself towards values-driven action instead of being driven by fear, anxiety, worry, or autopilot. You can respond rather than react. Recognising the stress response and being able to name the emotions you are experiencing and choose your response is emotional intelligence which we will look at in the next chapter.

> Your interpretation, the story you tell yourself, is critical to the emotion you experience and how much stress you feel.

## MINDFULNESS, THE STRESS RESPONSE AND TOLERATING DISCOMFORT

Mindfulness skills can help you to:

- name your stressors
- notice when your stress response is activated
- notice when you are amplifying pain and creating suffering
- name your emotions, values, beliefs and meaning
- make a different, more helpful choice.

The ability to pay attention in the present moment without judgement will help you notice what you are experiencing, including discomfort. Mindfulness asks you to stay present to *whatever* you are experiencing. To respond more effectively to stressors, you need to learn to tolerate discomfort. Be present to discomfort rather than avoiding or suppressing it.

Since you work in medicine, you have already decided at some level that you are willing to be in the presence of human suffering. Stressors are inherent in the work you do. Are you present to others' suffering but ignoring your own pain? When your stress response is activated, your fight or flight instincts would have you resist or run in order to be safe. Staying present to your own discomfort seems counterintuitive. What do you need so that you can *stay with* your own internal experiences?

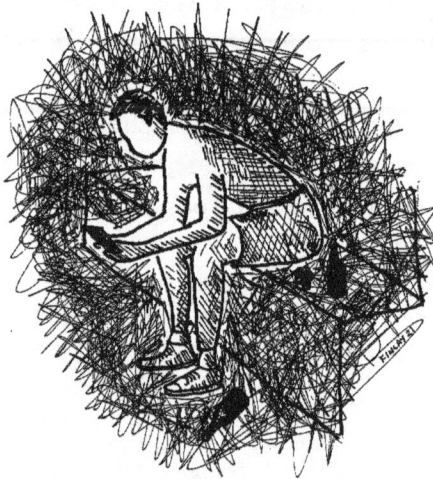

Rather than tolerating distress, humans distract and numb themselves with the quick fixes of drugs, alcohol, exercise, food, gaming, porn, endless scrolling through social media, keeping busy, etc. These distraction and avoidance tactics seem to work – in the short term. In fact, these behaviours are drawing you away from what you value most. They keep you in the red zone, trapped in sympathetic dominance, a vicious cycle that keeps you disengaged, disconnected, isolated and exhausted from what really matters. I have met many doctors who drink coffee in the morning to get going for the day, wine at night to help them sleep, and fill up every single spare moment of their days off with mindless busyness so as to drown out their inner critic.

# Coby's Story

*Coby is a successful, rapidly advancing, speciality surgeon. He worked very long hours in three hospitals in a major city. He was on several committees and was enjoying establishing himself as a go-to surgeon in his field. Coby came to coaching saying he needed better time management skills. His first child was just six months old, so uninterrupted sleep was a thing of the past. Coby was savvy, committed, and ambitious for himself, his family, and his patients. He was completely invested in being the best he could be.*

*When he wasn't thinking about work, he was on social media – he loved politics. One day as we were in session, he observed out loud that he was always on his phone, even when he was taking care of his young son. Later, he told me he liked to go for walks and would like to start running again like he had in his younger days. Then he paused, and realised he'd done neither for nearly a year.*

*Coaching had created enough space for Coby to notice his own behaviour. Of course, he knew about his habits already, but he hadn't taken enough space to really pause, to stop and notice their impact. He had avoided focusing on them. As coach, I held him to account by wanting to talk about what he was noticing, by not skating over his story. We stayed with these realities of his life as Coby felt his own discomfort about letting himself and his son down.*

*It's not easy work, those sessions were no doubt uncomfortable for him! Making the changes he decided to make in the following weeks was also uncomfortable, but what he achieved as a result was priceless – the relationships with his son and his wife that he wanted. As a result of feeling the discomfort and being clear about his values, Coby was able to recalibrate and find a more sustainable balance. He started thinking about energy rather than time, and he redirected some of his energy towards his family and health values. He was able to step into his discomfort in the safe container of coaching.*

In mindfulness, you stay present to what you feel and think, learning to tolerate distress and discomfort. You practise observing your experience with curiosity and acceptance, and allowing your emotions with compassion, patience, and kindness. As you tune into your body, learning to welcome all of your internal experiences, you can grow your capacity to take good care of yourself, even in stressful times.

> **Get comfortable with being uncomfortable.**

We will look at compassion more in Chapter 7, but I want to point to it specifically as an important part of responding effectively to stress. When your body activates its stress response, it does so for good reason; it believes there is a threat that you need to be aware of and be ready to respond to, principally by fighting or running away. The problem is that this same physiological response activates in the same way to perceived threats when there is no actual threat, keeping your body in a state of unnecessary arousal.

If you react to this red zone state with critical self-talk, impatience, and negativity, you maintain your higher levels of cortisol and adrenaline and you sling second arrows, amplifying the pain. You practise the habits of negativity and stress. Each time you strengthen the neurological pathways for these behaviours, you end up feeling exhausted, disempowered, and disenchanted. This reactive pattern is a downward spiral and a waste of your energy.

Self-compassion is the antidote to this pattern. Kristen Neff and Chris Gerber describe self-compassion as having three components:

1. Mindfulness – noticing what's happening
2. Recognising that you are human and suffer just like all humans do
3. Show yourself kindness, talk to yourself as you would a best friend

The opposite of these self-compassion qualities, according to Germer and Neff (2019), is self-judgement, isolation, and over-identification with the problems or the pain you have in your life. A doctor in this state seems only a short step away from burnout.

Remember Coby? As we brought our collective attention to his constant social media scrolling – constant even when spending time with his young son – we practised mindfulness and kindness. I did not judge him for his behaviour. Rather, I asked him with genuine curiosity what he was looking at on his phone, and what he liked about it.

In seeking to understand, a space was created for Coby to lean into. What he noticed was a gap between his behaviour and who he wanted to be as a father. Coby felt his own discomfort – these were moments of suffering. We recognised together how uncomfortable this was and how hard it is to be all the things we want to be. We recognised the challenges of living up to our own standards. Coby felt and observed his humanness. He made his changes grounded in self-compassion, knowing it would be difficult and he would need some support from his wife. Funnily enough, once he made his values-based decisions, his awareness was so heightened that it turned out to be easy! A month later, he told me lots of happy stories about his son and said he wasn't missing twitter at all.

Self-compassion is not soft and fluffy, it takes practice to build these skills and practising requires discipline. Nor is it self-pity, self-indulgence, or selfishness. Johnson and O'Brien found self-compassion to be associated with fewer negative states including stress, depression, anxiety, and shame. It is worth noting the research shows that people who practise self-compassion are:

- better able to cope with tough situations like divorce or chronic pain
- more compassionate toward others
- engaged in healthier habits like exercise.

Sometimes doctors see themselves as different to other people – you are not different when it comes to suffering. Holding this belief either explicitly or implicitly is a risk to your wellbeing, setting you up to expect only a life of ease, denying your humanity and the realities of the world or disconnecting you from other people. Accepting your human quality might even turn out to feel liberating.

> Believing you can withstand anything all the time for a long time is tantamount to saying you are not human.

I don't believe you are a robot. To keep doing your work as a doctor, you need to know how to look after yourself. Having skills in self-compassion means you can meet yourself in suffering and hold your own hand in those dark moments long enough to bear the pain. You can be with yourself with an open heart and a clear mind so that you can work your way through whatever is happening. Recover and heal, show up again in good shape, able to do your work without causing harm to anyone, including yourself. When you are able to do this for yourself, you are better able to do it with others, including your family.

Self-compassion doesn't have to take a long time, like most habits of wellbeing it's more important to practise a little bit often so that you feel cared for and loved often, and so that you strengthen these neurological pathways instead of the default pathways of suppression and avoidance. In self-compassion, you take a moment to honour what is here, and to acknowledge and respect your own effort, your human quality, and your need.

> Self-compassion is a balancing habit, one that can help restore the balance between your stress response and your relaxation response, changing your neurochemistry, self-talk, thoughts, and emotions.

## SIX HABITS TO HELP YOU LIVE MORE IN THE GREEN ZONE

Habits are patterns that help your brain conserve energy. Small routines that you repeat regularly can help or hinder your wellbeing. For instance, getting only erratic sleep and smoking cigarettes can erode your wellbeing and your performance. Drinking water regularly throughout the day and going for a daily 20-minute walk can enhance your wellbeing and performance.

It is not my aim here to construct your healthy habits for you, but to acknowledge that every tiny thing you do makes a difference to how you relate to your inner and outer world. Each time you repeat a behaviour, you strengthen your neurological pathways for that habit. Over time, it gets easier to repeat. Your brain is built for it, you build the pathways unwittingly or on purpose. Either way, you are building neurological pathways that determine your behaviour, your thinking, your emotions, and your life.

> Be careful what you cultivate, because what you cultivate becomes your life.

When you cultivate your self-awareness, attention, and regulation, your capacity to notice when you move away from your values and when your beliefs are hindering you is increased. When you are able to do this, you are more attuned to what is causing you stress and you can intervene, helping you to spend more of the time in the green zone and less in the red zone. If you want to learn, grow, change, develop, or help others to do so, you will want to be living in the green zone much more often. Here are six conscious practices to help you cultivate better balance.

## 1. Get enough good-quality sleep

As a doctor on call or working shifts, your sleep can take a serious hit in terms of both quantity and quality. Research consistently shows that adults need between 7 and 9 hours of sleep every night, and that the best way to support your wellbeing is to have these hours of sleep in a routine way about the same time every night. People who sleep well have longer lifespans and better health.

When that is not possible, consider building a 10- to 20-minute power nap into your day. Research from John Hopkins suggests that adults who nap between 1pm and 4pm benefit cognitively. If you need more recovery sleep, nap for 90 minutes so that you move through a full sleep cycle. The sleep foundation suggests that napping in this way can improve learning, aid memory formation, and regulate emotions. Refer to Chapter 3 for more information on sleep.

## 2. Remember you are not your thoughts

Human beings are meaning-making creatures who use stories to explain the world. Your stories are filled with what matters and biasedly ignore much of the detail. Your brain is biased towards the negative because negative factors threaten your survival the most, so they are the most important things to remember.

If you find yourself in an ambiguous situation – let's say your consultant told you to be more empathic or to 'behave more like a consultant' – you may not know what to do. In this example, the feedback is not specific enough, so your brain will err on the negative side just in case, ensuring your safety. As a result, your confidence is likely to take a hit because your brain is leaning towards a negative interpretation, even if the consultant only said it as a passing comment and then forgot about it herself the next day. There is a perceived danger here that may or may not be real, but while it is uncertain your brain will consider it as dangerous.

> The story you tell yourself can help or hinder you.

If you are telling yourself a story about not being good enough, remember that medicine has fostered cultural beliefs about being perfect, resilient, and achieving at all costs. These stories are not necessarily helpful. These stories induce enormous amounts of suffering, amplify pain, and activate the stress response, keeping you in the red zone much more than you need to be. Let go of your unhelpful stories. You are the thinker of your thoughts, hold them lightly and look for thoughts that serve you better.

Enquire if there is another story. You don't need to be welded on to a thought just because your brain offered it. Practise saying to yourself *that's an interesting story, I wonder what other stories there are*, and even *thank you mind for that story, I'm not going with that one today*. Be a bit circumspect with your stories, they may or may not be true. Even if they are true, ask, *is this serving me*? Learn to detach from your thoughts and to use a wider lens, this will help you stay in the green zone more, where you can learn, grow, and heal much more readily.

# ACTIVITY 10

**Try this**

Take a pen and hold it in a tight fist, hold onto it as tightly as you can. Keep holding it for the next minute or two. Is your hand getting tired? Are you distracted by the exercise? Maybe you are having some thoughts about the pen or the exercise. Maybe you are starting to wonder what the point of this is. As your mind wanders, your muscles might cramp and you might start to feel annoyed, perhaps you even notice that your stress response is activated.

Take a break, release the pen and hold it now on your open palm. I'm guessing that feels a little easier. You could probably sit like this for quite a long time. Just as you hold your pen lightly, see if you can hold your stories lightly too. They might be true; they might not be true. This circumspect approach allows you to see clearly and lets you practise more psychological flexibility. You are more creative and more able to choose your response from here. Practise approaching your stories about stress with curiosity, accept that there are other possible descriptions and hold all your stories lightly.

## 3. Reframe time

More than half of the doctors I meet tell me they need to learn how to manage their time better. Perhaps you've said this too.

> Stop focusing on time, which is finite, and start focusing on energy.

Unlike time, energy can be influenced by you. Some activities leave you feeling depleted, and some energise you. Start noticing which activities and people energise you and choose how you want to spend your time based on energy.

Try another word experiment by replacing the word *time* with the word *energy:*

→     I don't have enough time to go to that meeting... I don't have enough *energy* for that meeting

→     I ran out of time to finish my file notes this morning... I ran out of *energy* to finish my file notes this morning

→     There wasn't enough time to talk further with the patient on the ward round... There wasn't enough *energy* to talk further with the patient on the ward round

> **Every time you hear yourself saying I don't have enough time, replace the word with energy and see what the impact is.**

We feel stress when our capacity is reaching its limits – not enough time, appointments, bandages, nurses, theatre lists, hours in the day. This also applies to our internal capacity.

Each time you bring your consciousness to a word, you challenge the idea and make a space big enough to notice something new, to detach a little from it and to see it clearly. You may decide to keep it exactly as it was before. At least you are choosing now instead of defaulting reactively, living in the red zone, feeling out of control or stressed out. Be accountable, at least to yourself. If you decided not to go to the meeting because it's not a productive use of your time, be honest about that to yourself. Recognise that you are choosing to prioritise how you use your resources – your energy and your time. This is personal agency at work in service of what you believe and value. You are living on purpose, creating the conditions you need to thrive.

## 4. Be proactive

Stephen R. Covey wrote a best-selling book in 1989 called *'The 7 Habits of Highly Effective People'*. He called the first habit *'Be Proactive,'* which is about self-awareness. He reflected on Victor Frankl's wisdom and noticed the gap between stimulus and response, and he noticed what Frankl said about the gap – this is where we have freedom to choose. Covey also noticed that proactive people accept what he called *response-ability*, and they make values-based decisions.

There are two important ideas Covey reminds us of in his *Be Proactive* habit. The first is to listen to our language: is your language proactive or reactive? Do you take responsibility for your circumstances and focus on what you can control and influence, or do you have the habits of blame, deflect, and distract?

Asking you to describe your body as *activated* instead of *stressed* is an example of experimenting with the impact of language. Previously I asked you to replace *should* with *could*, suggesting you move from a reactive word of obligation to a proactive value-based word. Just now I invited you to be accountable about your priorities when you think about your time and energy. These conscious changes are helping to raise the awareness you have around where you put your effort.

The second idea Covey shared that can help you respond more effectively to stress is to ask yourself if what you are occupying your mind and body with is within your circle of concern or your circle of influence. Your circle of concern is probably large. It might include concern about the environment, politics, healthcare, education, and many other things. Within that large circle, you likely have some more specific concerns: your actual patients, your own children's education or your bank balance for example. This smaller circle is your circle of influence, these are things you can actually do something about and where you should spend most of your energy and time.

Reactive people focus their attention on their circle of concern, noticing other people's behaviour and blaming systemic weaknesses. This has the impact of reducing their circle of influence, leaving them feeling disempowered. Proactive people are aware of where their influence lies and spend their effort there, because when they do, they enlarge and magnify their impact, increasing their circle of influence over time.

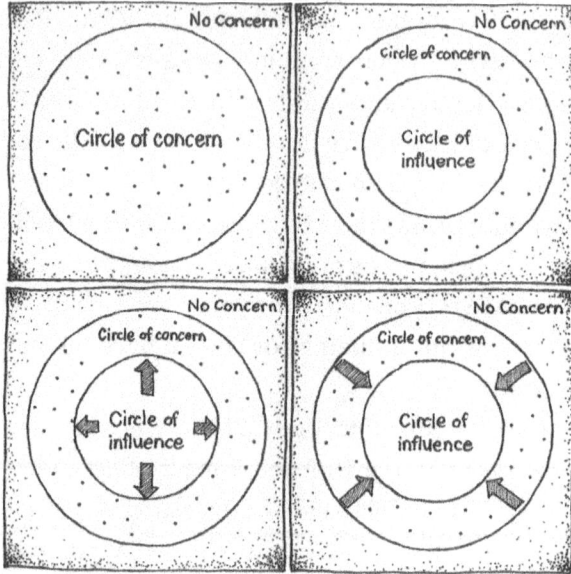

Professor Catherine Crock understood this when she started the Hush Foundation 20 years ago. At that time, she wanted to help the families she worked with at Melbourne's Royal Children's Hospital have a better experience. Cath works as a haematologist; her patients are children with cancer. She wanted to understand how their experience of coming into theatre for a lumber puncture could be made less frightening. Cath started her work in the area she had some influence – in her ward with her team of colleagues and their patients.

The Hush Foundation's work is now felt all around the world through their arts programs, sharing beautiful music produced for hospitals and the Gathering of Kindness movement aimed at cultivating kinder workplaces for healthcare workers. Cath and the Hush Foundation have expanded their circle of influence continuously as in the bottom left figure in Covey's model, by keeping their focus on what they could influence.

Focusing on your circle of influence and engaging proactively and responsibly within that will grow your influence and agency in the long run, empowering you in your own life and helping you feel more able to respond effectively to the stressors in your life.

> Give your mental and physical energy, time, and effort to those things you can actually influence. You will have more impact and reduce your negative stress.

## 5. Practise self-compassion

When doctors hear about self-compassion as an antidote to stress, they can be dismissive. It sounds too soft and fluffy perhaps, completely counterintuitive to the medical culture of harden up, compete, and do it perfectly.

> Doctors often behave like they are allergic to self-compassion.

Many doctors have told me they exhaust their compassion budget at work and don't have much left when they get home for themselves or their families.

What is it you value most of all? When you worked through Activity 4 in Chapter 4, what did you name as the thing that matters most to you? If you said your health or your family, then there is something wrong with this picture of living in the red zone most of the time and resisting self-compassion.

Some of your stress is coming from not living in a way that is true to your values. If you truly value your health and your family, what can you do today to honour these values? To make a course correction, consider these questions:

- Would you like to show yourself more compassion?
- How about your family?
- Out of 10, how important is it to you?

Define your intention, you can start practising as soon as you are ready. Make one small decision about what action you can take today to show some compassion to yourself.

---

## ACTIVITY 11

### Self-Compassion Practice

**Try this – allow about five minutes**

This is a mindful practice for self-compassion.

- Sit comfortably in your chair with your feet on the floor and eyes closed.
- Notice your body, gently scan up and down your body for a minute or two.
- No need for criticism or judgement, simply check in with your physical body, enquiring with gentle curiosity – how are you?
- Now bring your attention to your breath, settle your awareness here and observe the inhalation and the exhalation for a few breaths as a neutral observer.
- For a few moments, call to mind a current situation in your life that you are resisting, something unwanted that you might wish was otherwise.
- When you call to mind this situation, what do you feel in your body? Do you notice tension or any discomfort that you can describe?
- Notice the discomfort or tension for a few moments and let it be in your body without commentary or criticism.
- Now acknowledge to yourself that you are human and you are responding to a challenge, you might like to notice your body's appropriate activation.
- Now gently say something kind to yourself, something you might say to a dear friend like, *hang in there, you are doing the best you can,* or *it's good to sit with this for a few moments to understand it some more.*
- When you are ready, open your eyes, stretch your body and smile to yourself for taking the time to notice yourself.

### 6. Practise Gratitude

Practising gratitude regularly is a great way to balance the heavy load you may have on one end of your seesaw. There is a depth of research supporting the impact these practices have on our wellbeing. You may have come to know the stressors in your life intimately. If that is all you focus on, you are keeping all your weight on one end of the seesaw. To bring some balance to your mental health, make a simple gratitude practice every day for a month and observe whatever you experience.

---

## ACTIVITY 12

### Gratitude

Choose one time in the day. This could be as you wake up or as you go to bed, at dinner with your family, as you arrive home each day or when you write in your journal. Sit for a minute quietly, feel into your body, check in with yourself. Now write or say out loud one to three things that you are grateful for today.

I am grateful that you are taking some time to prioritise taking care of yourself by building skills and practising. Thank you.

---

## SUMMARY

Being specific about the stressors in your life will help you take effective action to change things for the better. Living in the red zone of chronic stress damages your physical and mental health and prevents you from being a truly great doctor. The way you think about stressors in your life can amplify them and do more damage than the original trigger.

There is no exact recipe for responding to stressors more effectively as a doctor. Here are a few key behaviours that will help you live in the green zone more. Choose one to start with and practise. After a few weeks, add another habit to consciously practise.

## Actions for reducing stress

- Pay attention to your sleep, prioritise routines that create good quality sleep for at least seven hours a night. If you are not shift working, get up at about the same time every day.
- Cultivate a different relationship with stress. Raise your awareness, learn how to recognise the specific stressor. Recognise that most stressors cause short-term activation, you choose to extend it.
- Try saying '*my body is activated*' instead of saying you're stressed. Be specific about what it is activating to.
- Name and notice when you are in the red and the green zones. Choose one habit to help you come back into the green zone and commit to practising it regularly.
- Learn the skills of mindfulness and self-compassion. Be proactive, find a coach or peer to help you maintain your practice and embed helpful habits.
- Work within your circle of influence. As you meet your real needs, reframe your experience, use your energy only on what you can control.
- Get comfortable with being uncomfortable, lean into your learning edge.
- Practise gratitude every day.

# 6

# EMOTIONAL INTELLIGENCE AND AGILITY

*"One ought to hold onto one's heart: for if one lets it go,*
*one soon loses control of the head too."*
*— Fredrich Nietzsche*

In this chapter, we will take some time to understand emotions. Then I will walk you through how you can apply the knowledge and practices in this book to three specific emotions that your colleagues regularly bring to coaching – anxiety, guilt, and shame. Thriving means being able to respond to everything life brings you, to meet your experiences confident in your capacity and fluency, it does not mean an easy life.

Medicine has actively taught you to avoid expression of emotions. Emotions have been treated as a vulnerability to be avoided in order to do good medicine. Essentially, emotions have been treated like a small child playing peek-a-boo; if you don't mention them and you can't see them, they don't exist. Your expression of your emotions at work has not been welcomed but, as you know, they certainly exist.

Countless doctors have told me stories of being off work sick and not a single colleague phoning them to ask them if they are ok. On their return to work it has been the same – no one asks. As a human being, you have a deeply rooted need to be seen and heard. When you are not, you feel it. As we have seen in Chapter 4, this artificial separation of your role as doctor from your *self* is difficult to sustain, unnecessary, and unrealistic.

Worse than being ignored, some doctors even accuse each other of being emotional as if it is a demeaning insult. A stunning example of this was shared by Dr Yumiko Kadota in her memoir, when she described being denigrated by a male registrar at 3am in the morning. Rather than apologise or rethink, he claimed the protocol required it and told her to "Calm down, you're being an emotional female". This is a story that has resonated across the globe with female doctors.

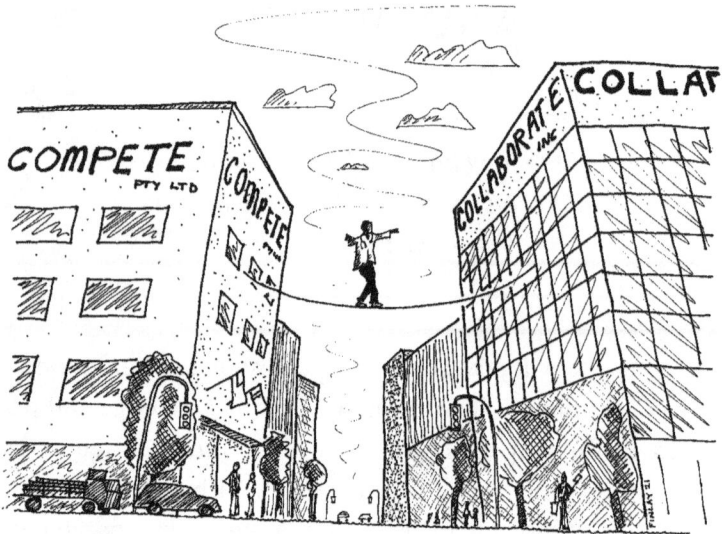

In medicine, you walk a tightrope of competing and collaborating, supporting each other at the same time as competing for training, jobs, research grants, status, referrals. All of this by itself creates a hotbed of emotions. Let's name them and learn how to work with them rather than pretending they are not here.

## DOCTORS AND RATIONAL THOUGHT

The prevailing story inside medicine is that emotions interfere with rational thought and good medicine. This artificial separation of rational and emotional thought is unhelpful, inaccurate, and out of date in terms of how we understand human thinking and behaviour.

Psychologists and neurologists have shown us that emotions are complex and involved in every single experience and decision in our lives. As the research becomes more sophisticated, the idea of rational thinking and intuitive or emotional thinking being separate has been shown to be a flawed idea. Your brain is primed to build intricate circuits that are designed for survival using all the data it can gather, including emotional data.

As Jerome Groopman MD writes in his book 'How Doctors Think', "Most errors are mistakes in thinking. And part of what causes these cognitive errors is our inner feelings, feelings we do not readily admit to and often don't even recognise". He goes on to describe this as a paradox, saying that "Feeling prevents us from being blind to our patient's soul but risks blinding us to what is wrong with him". Without an ability to notice your emotions and use them intelligently, you are more open to using stereotypes and attribution error to understand the world. To become immune to the emotions your work naturally evokes is to diminish your role, Groopman says, from *healer* to *tactician.*

Skilfully engaging with your emotions is a powerful way for you to flourish, to be effective in your relationships, to be well in your internal world and to deliver your best performance as a doctor. Learn about them, understand them and work with them, rather than suppressing, denying, or struggling with them.

## EMOTIONAL INTELLIGENCE

Using the energy of your emotions well for your own experience in life and for when you are seeking to persuade and influence others is emotional intelligence. Without these skills, emotions can get in your way, sapping your energy, sabotaging your intention, and creating conflict.

Self-awareness, effective stress management, an ability to regulate your thoughts, understanding bias, and being present will go a long way towards a better medical life, but without emotional intelligence you are like a ship with a loose rudder.

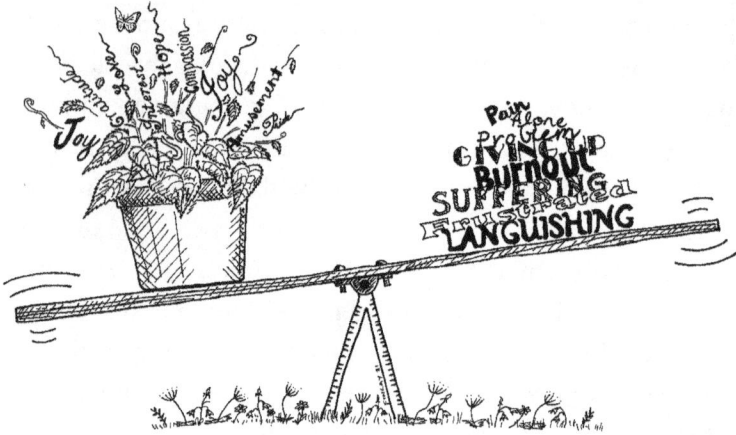

Remember the active elements of a person who is flourishing: PERMA. The first element is positive emotions: hope, interest, joy, love, compassion, pride, gratitude, amusement. These emotions promote well-being and can undo the harmful effects of what we think of as negative emotions. The more of these you have on the other end of your seesaw, the more balance you can achieve in your life. You can build positive emotions by:

- Spending time with people you care about
- Doing activities you love
- Listening to uplifting music
- Being outside in nature
- Reflecting on what you are grateful for
- Exercising
- Contemplation practice

The other elements of PERMA – engagement (flow), strong support-ive relationships, meaning, accomplishments – have positive emotional content. Flourishers work *with* rather than *against* their emotions. For you to truly flourish and have agency in your own life, you need to be able to work with your emotions and those of others.

Understanding your own emotional data will allow you to take proactive action, meeting your own needs earlier. Accurately understanding the emotional data coming from others more often means you can build stronger connections with them and are more consistently able to avoid conflict. In other words, you are better able to take care of yourself and others.

The key is in learning how to use your emotions intelligently to understand your own needs and those of others in real time. Emotions have evolved as a means to help humans connect and bond for our survival. They are central to empathy and compassion too, which are necessary skills for providing excellent healthcare. We will look at empathy and compassion in the next chapter.

> Researchers have found that the more accurately you interpret your own emotions, the better you are at interpreting and understanding other people's emotions.

When it comes to emotions, you need skills on two fronts. Consciously commit to prioritising activities that generate positive emotions more often in your life. And learn how to respond more effectively to the emotions that you might think of as negative or overwhelming, which is what this chapter aims to help you do.

## EMOTIONAL AGILITY

Emotional agility is being able to recognise your emotions in real time, using the gap between stimulus and response to *choose how* you respond. Being emotionally agile means that you can orient to more useful responses when things change, rather than reacting in ways that bring negativity or are unhelpful. Emotionally agile people are psychologically flexible and able to respond to complexity and uncertainty more readily. They are less likely to get stuck in their existing cognitive templates (their habits). In your healthcare environment, these skills can make a world of difference to your effectiveness and your wellbeing.

## Aya's Story

*Aya works as an obstetrician and gynaecologist. She teaches lots of trainees and is heavily invested in their development as people. She told me her job in surgery is inherently risky and there are lots of things that can go wrong. She described being able to concentrate as her most essential skill and said that this was much easier when the theatre environment was safe and people trusted each other.*

*Aya came to coaching five years ago after receiving feedback that she was too blunt in her communication with her colleagues, especially the junior doctors. The feedback Aya received about being blunt was painful. Yet after her initial introspective crisis, she met the feedback with the intention to learn. It has taken a concerted effort over time, but she has learnt to work intelligently with her emotions and as a result she has changed her experience at work.*

*In our sessions, Aya has focused specifically on growing her own emotional literacy so she can be more emotionally agile in her work. Aya says that the culture of medicine implies that it's okay to talk about patient emotions, but not to talk about your own emotions, especially as a female surgeon. Yet the more she has named emotion and responded to other's emotions with empathy and curiosity, the more connected she has felt to her colleagues.*

*As a result of her focused long-term effort, she has built an entirely different reputation to the one she was establishing before the feedback. Now she says it's never been easier for her to concentrate in theatre, she feels psychologically safe and she believes her team does too. She has led her team to learn about emotions by implicit example and explicit teaching. She has supported herself by maintaining her coaching and being willing to be vulnerable and to experiment. Learning about her emotions has made a huge difference for Aya, and the impact has rippled out to her team. She now believes that medicine misled her about the impact of emotions in her work.*

## SO WHAT IS AN EMOTION ANYWAY?

> Universal primary emotions are here for a reason, they are survival imperatives.

Psychologist Dr Paul Ekman has studied emotion since 1954, seeking to understand what the primary human emotions are and trying to determine if they have universal facial expressions that are recognised across cultures. He has concluded that there are six primary emotions shared by all people across the world: anger, surprise, disgust, enjoyment, fear, and sadness. He says there is strong evidence for a seventh emotion too: contempt.

We categorise emotions like happiness or excitement as positive, and those like sadness or anger as negative. This binary thinking is not helpful when it comes to our emotional wellbeing, because it suggests that there is something wrong or bad about most possible emotions. Look at Ekman's universal basic emotions, only one – enjoyment – would be classed as necessarily positive. Surprise could go either way, and the remaining five would be considered negative. Yet each emotion has evolved in us for a reason. Evolution has promoted the factors that are helpful to your survival.

Fear, anxiety, and disgust are powerful emotions that can feel very uncomfortable, but they keep us safe, they are obvious protectors. The most uncomfortable emotions, shame and guilt, are here to keep us safe too, because they help us behave in ways that make us acceptable to our group. They encourage us to comply with social norms.

> All primary emotions are central to your key survival tactic, they exist to help you stay in the group.

What happens in your thinking when you consider all of your emotions as neutral? What would happen if you could welcome all emotions as integral to your life, helping you perform better and connect more, rather than keeping you quiet and feeling bad? My invitation to you is to start experimenting with the idea that *every* emotion is here for a reason, and that reason is to keep you alive. Welcome all of them, be curious and seek to learn from them.

> Welcome your emotions and hold them lightly with curiosity and compassion. Be courageous enough to want to know yourself.

Focusing on your technical or clinical medical skills, only working with your so-called rational brain, parking your emotions at the door in the name of professionalism when you arrive at work, is like working with one hand tied behind your back. Sure, you can become quite adept working with one hand, but why would you want to when you have two? Two hands are so much more efficient and effective than one.

Your mind is interpreting all the possible data to predict the world and your safety in it 24/7, but the brain makes many different minds. The one universal thing your brain and everyone else's brain does is produce affect all of the time, whether you are aware of it or not. Your affect is like a barometer letting you and others know how you are doing. Neuroscientists agree that affect demonstrates that your body is biologically a part of your mind. What they do not yet agree on is what makes you feel pleasant, unpleasant, calm, or agitated. Why do we feel differently? The answer so far is that your brain creates your own social reality and that is not the same as mine or anyone else's.

> The emotions you feel cause physiological responses that you then seek to explain with your thoughts.

Have you ever met someone you instantly didn't like or didn't trust? That's your unconscious brain making a prediction outside of your awareness and telling you via your body and your emotions to be careful. You don't need to know all the pros and cons about whether you *should* like the person, your body tells you within a few seconds. If you are tuning in, you adjust your behaviour accordingly and hold back.

Sometime later, your conscious thinking mind gets involved, but it might not be much use. It's likely your thoughts will be something like, *I don't know, I just didn't warm to her.* You are cognitively attempting to explain what happened after the event. Your body-mind already 'did' the emotions.

> **Your body and your emotions act as signposts to understand the world, and they activate instantly without conscious thought.**

Imagine you are in clinic, it's busy, and you are double booked. The patient you are currently with has just burst into tears and disclosed to you that their partner has abused them. This is only the second time you have met the patient.

**What happens in your body in this moment?**

Did you answer this question with a thought? Something like:

- *Oh no, not today, there is no time, I'm already running late.*
- *Why me? I'm not a social worker!*
- *There goes my chance of getting home on time...*
- *Thank goodness she told someone, no wonder her affect is so low.*

All these thoughts are common and normal. The first three reflect the resistance I talked about in Chapter 5 that people experience all the time. These are all thoughts. Take another look at the question. **What happened in your *body*?**

If you don't know, it's a good place to start enquiring into. Build your emotional literacy by noticing your body. Name what you are feeling with a sensations word (e.g. hot) and then enquire if there is an emotion with that sensation that you can name (there won't always be, sometimes it's just a hot day). Being curious raises your internal awareness.

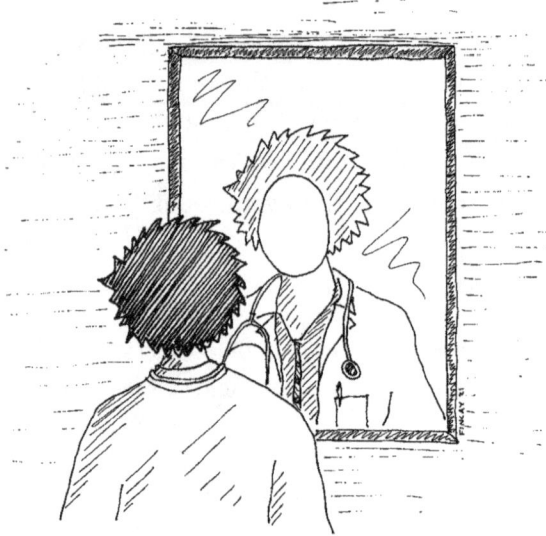

If you noticed your posture change to be more upright or more slumped, that will tell you something about your emotional response too. You might have noticed a tightness in your jaw, stomach, or shoulders. These body shifts signpost various emotions. The change in your body might have indicated anger, concern, feelings of protectiveness, weariness, or something else. Noticing your emotions in real time allows you to make different choices over time, better choices.

> In the western world, we sometimes define emotions as the opposite of rational thinking. This is a mistake because the right emotional response can be entirely rational.

Imagine you are out for a run by yourself in the bush when you meet a venomous Australian snake, who rears up as if to strike when you are three steps away from it and travelling fast. Your emotional reaction of fear induces you to pivot mid-air and run off the other way faster than you thought possible. Your body and emotions caused this reaction using your unconscious thinking. And it was entirely rational, given the circumstances.

This *emotion* of fear triggered physiological changes, *sensations you could feel,* like a raised heart rate, faster breathing, and powerful legs. You *feel y*our emotions. They are generated by your predicting brain, born out of your social reality and cognitive templates.

The snake gave you a fright. As well as feeling fear, you may have also experienced surprise because you saw the snake when you were almost standing on it. If you have never seen a snake in the wild before, you might respond differently to it, compared to if you had met lots of snakes out running in the bush. Depending on your unique history and affect, when you arrive home safely you might think *that was lucky,* or you might burst into tears and decide to never go running in the bush again. Your thoughts and emotions arise from *your* particular social reality, they are a unique combination for you. If you thought you were lucky, you might not understand the person who vows to never go again, and vice versa.

After the event, your mind uses your experience of meeting a snake in the bush to predict the world. Your experience is the foundation for future predictions about the world – thoughts (conscious and unconscious) that trigger emotions and physiological sensations.

> Emotions are in your whole body.

Your emotions are embodied responses to the world, a natural guidance system. You can think of them as signposts, but they are not always reliable, so they can cause confusion for you and for others.

The good news is, you can choose how you respond by learning how to expand the space between the stimulus and the response. As Lisa Feldman Barrett says in her book '*Seven and a Half Lessons About the Brain'*, even when you can't control the heat of the moment, you can change your predictions *before* the heat of the moment by making some automatic behaviours more likely than others.

> Your life becomes what you cultivate.

## HOW TO DEFUSE YOUR EMOTIONS

### ACTIVITY 13

### Defusing emotion

If all this noticing and naming is making you too uncomfortable, try this little hack to defuse the emotion and gain some clarity. Notice how your body feels, give the sensations an emotional name, say your emotions out loud to someone you trust, the dog, or even to yourself.

Instead of saying 'I'm relaxed', say, 'I'm *noticing* that I am relaxed'. Instead of saying 'I'm anxious's say, *'Anxiety is here'*.

Now you can look *at* the emotion instead of being *in* the emotion, you have created a little bit of distance. You are defusing.

Does it make a difference to how you feel and think? Remember to practise. Saying you are noticing something, or something is here, creates more awareness of the gap between stimulus and response. It separates you as distinct from what you are experiencing.

You can defuse your thoughts in this way too:

I'm having the thought that I am not good enough.
I notice my brain is making a story about being an imposter.

You are not your thought; you are *having* a thought or an emotion.

## USING THE GAP BETWEEN STIMULUS AND RESPONSE TO YOUR ADVANTAGE

Your 'hot' brain is another way of describing your stress response, and usually refers to negative emotions with high energy like anger and rage. If you have a situation at work that triggers your fight or flight response, like a difficult relationship with a colleague, you are already primed to expect challenges and the emotional upset that comes with them. In this circumstance, you cannot think straight. Your prefrontal cortex goes offline, and the alarm centres of your brain activate your mind and body. This means that the decision-making part of your brain has checked out temporarily. In the heat of the moment, it is impossible to craft a plan. You need a pre-determined plan that you have tried, tested and practised.

A pre-determined plan is simple, and aims to slow things down so that you respond rather than react with a default pattern:

1. Take a breath, ideally a long exhalation.
2. Identify what's happening inside yourself. Do this in the third person giving the feeling a name – 'anger is here' (not 'I am angry').
3. Naming the emotion in the third person creates a tiny space, a feeling of distance between the stimulus and the response. Now you are looking at the situation instead of from it.
4. You have reminded yourself that there is a choice of responses. You can defuse a little.
5. Adjust your body to generate a sense of control – feel your feet on the floor or stand up a little straighter.

As you name the experience – anger is here – you tune into your breath. You may not be able to take the long exhale right there, you might look like you are sighing in exasperation (not a good move). However, internally tuning into your breath, just observing it, even for only two or three seconds, slows everything in your mind and body down and gives your prefrontal cortex a chance to re-engage. If you have been practising mindfulness in some way, you will have strengthened the connections between your prefrontal cortex neurons and the amygdala, the alarm centre of your brain. Over time you will get better at this kind of regulation because your neuronal pathway will develop from a dirt track into a highway, and the messages will have an easier, smoother transmission.

# Greg's Story

*Greg works as an ENT surgeon and came to me for help regarding his interactions with colleagues. There had been several occasions over a period of six months where another surgeon had questioned his decisions publicly, in both meetings and hallway conversations. Each time it happened, Greg had felt defensive and shown his anger, arguing with his colleague. He knew he looked disagreeable and worried that people had started to avoid him. He was angry with the other surgeon for causing the problem and anxious about his reputation, which he thought had been unfairly tarnished.*

*I challenged Greg to focus on what he could do to mitigate future conflicts, rather than relying on a change in behaviour from the other surgeon. Greg needed to practise his response to these situations before he got into the next one so that he would be able to respond differently in the heat of the moment. It was no good waiting until the next confrontation with the other surgeon to try a new response, because his automated response would kick in before he realised.* **To create an opportunity to respond differently, he had to train.**

*The key skill he trained was to feel his body and pause. In these few seconds of slowing down, he gave himself the opportunity to get in front of his automated reactions. He learnt to lengthen the gap between the stimulus and the response by simply taking one breath before he said anything. In the gap, he imagined one drum beat, and he noticed his emotion by checking his body. If there was tension, tightness, or heat, he decided he would not speak in front of others. He would ask his surgeon colleague to confer off to the side. He also sought a separate conversation with his colleague on the phone, to try to resolve what the real issue was.*

You don't need to do this conscious processing all day long for every interaction you have, but the more often you do it, the more opportunity you give yourself to respond to emotion intelligently. You increase your skill for the next time you are in the heat of the moment. You are learning and practising to defuse, manage, and regulate your emotions. Suppressing and denying emotion is more akin to gathering up more burden to carry around. This is emotional labour.

> **Different emotions activate different physiology,
> your response is a choice.**

To understand and work with your emotions, you need to be able to interpret your body signals and describe them with language. We started this work of emotional literacy back in Chapter 3, when we were thinking about self-regulation. For practice, notice your body in this moment. Take a long slow breath and see if you can name the physiological feelings (sensations) you have, and the emotions they might be signposting.

You might notice your temperature, tension, or mood. Perhaps you have tingling in your toes from pins and needles, maybe you have a sore back from gardening, or playing hockey, or standing in theatre all day. Maybe you notice that you are frowning. Your physical body can help you identify the emotion you are currently experiencing. Perhaps your sore back indicates tiredness, stress, frustration, or defensiveness. Maybe you are frowning because you are concentrating or confused by what you are reading.

> **Emotional responses are embedded in all your experiences, and your
> physiology can help you name them.**

Lisa Feldman-Barratt is one of the world's leading researchers into how we create emotion. She and her colleagues have found that, other than a few very simple emotional reactions that are present in babies, our emotions come about because of the way our brain makes guesses and predictions about the environment that are meaningful to us. It's these predictions and guesses that generate emotion. We generate different emotions from the same triggers because we interpret them differently. We then remember these experiences – the emotions and the memories – and use them for future predictions.

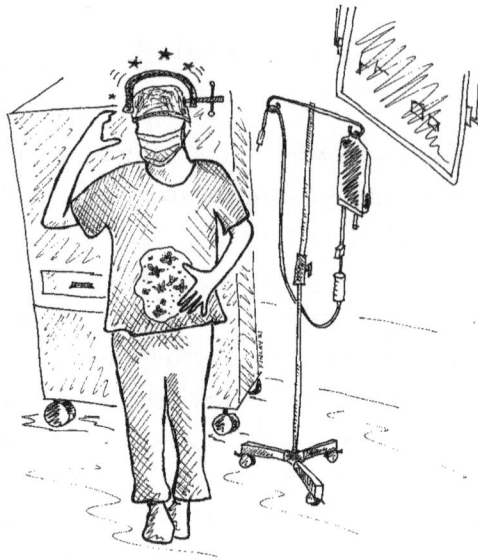

Emotions occur in response to stimuli – real, perceived and imagined. Although emotions have consistent and unique physiological markers, they are not the same in everyone. For example, you might feel anxious about speaking to your peers at a conference and experience your anxiety with an upset stomach. Your colleague who also feels anxious might break out in a red rash on his neck.

Every day, you make thousands of small and large decisions. All of them include a combination of emotion and cognition, most of which you are oblivious to. Your brain's 128 billion neurons communicate constantly, making meaning of your sensory data, and this complexity gives you the potential to be highly flexible in your responses.

> Learning what your emotions feel like in your body and what sort of energy they have, and giving these sensations names and understanding what triggers them, will give you many more response options.

The body sensations that signal emotion can be hard to describe sometimes. One way to describe them is through metaphor. A lack of progress that feels frustrating might be described as dragging your feet through the mud; feeling happy is walking on sunshine. In some instances, metaphor is more useful than naming the emotion because metaphor is a normal currency already in use in medicine. You should note that metaphor is culturally sensitive and may not be meaningful to other people.

> When you know how to understand and use emotions effectively, you will be more successful in all of your relationships – at home, at work with your patients and colleagues, and out in the wider world.

See if you can remember a time in your life when you thought something wasn't fair. Perhaps you noticed how many night shifts you had compared to your colleagues, and you heard yourself saying something like, "They take advantage of my good nature just because I haven't got kids". If you are feeling lonely and depleted, it's a short cognitive step to other thoughts like, "Why does this always happen to me?" and, "It's my fault for never speaking up, I'm weak" or, "They don't care about me".

These thoughts might be accompanied by emotions like sadness, shame or frustration. Without the capacity to notice these automatic thoughts and emotions, you are sliding down the same old slippery neurological pathway you've been on before. To have a different experience in your life, you need to first notice the hook and then be able to get off it.

You can use your diagnostic tools well because someone taught you. You have learnt through practice and making some mistakes. Perhaps you have had to seek guidance or advice from others to be truly skilled at using your diagnostic tools. Sometimes differential diagnosis has been complex. Perhaps there have been symptoms that have confused a clear outcome, creating dilemmas for you.

Bring all of this to deepening your learning about emotions. You will make some mistakes and you might need some help, it's the same as any other skill you have learnt. There are nuances and complexities. Sometimes even opposite emotions are present at the same time, causing confusion. For example, we often have happy-sad moments: finishing school and leaving the security of long-held friendships can be happy-sad, sharing a fond memory of a person who has died can be happy-sad, passing an exam and finding out your friend did not can be happy-sad, seeing a colleague off to a better job and reconciling that they won't be in your workplace with you any more can be happy-sad.

Emotions can be tricky to sort out and interpret, but don't let that deter you. Just as you have persisted in learning the nuances of your job so that you can provide better patient care and patient outcomes, learning the nuances of emotions can also help you provide better care of yourself and of your patients. As you learn to work intelligently with your emotions, you raise your capacity to take better care of yourself and to interact in relationships with others more effectively. This means you can become more influential and have greater impact, building high-trust connections and psychological safety into your environment.

> High-trust teams share their emotions. One of the great benefits of high-trust teams is how efficient they can become, ultimately saving everyone time, a commodity most doctors wish for.

Each time you notice an emotion in your body, practise giving it a name. The very act of pausing long enough to name the experience will help it progress. To respond effectively to any experience, we need to recognise it, to name it. Name it to tame it. Emotions are dynamic, name them and let them keep moving.

## EMOTIONS AND MEMORY, THE NEGATIVITY BIAS OF THE BRAIN

Our brains are intricately wired to be efficient and effective at keeping us alive, so your neurological emotional network and your memory network are intimately connected. To help you remember the right things to keep you safe, your body is wired to have intense emotions for the biggest threats to your survival and for these to be easily accessed from memory for future predictions.

If you learnt as a junior doctor that asking a question was risky, it is likely that you have stopped asking questions of your seniors unless you really have to. If you felt humiliated or embarrassed at a patient's bedside by the way a consultant spoke to you, that feeling is probably still very available to you. Perhaps you can even feel it in your body right now.

The emotion is directing your behaviour, limiting your learning, and causing your brain to keep predicting that the consultant you are with now should not be asked a question because it's too risky. In other words, you have taken a specific experience and generalised it to understand the world. Your experience of the world is determined by the old experience, the emotions related to it, and your narrowed attention in this situation. This is how your brain keeps you safe.

We are naturally attuned to the experiences that threaten our survival, they are automatically given our attention and our brain then predicts what could happen to keep us safe based on what it has learnt and remembered so far. The experiences are locked down into your brain and body by fast-acting chemistry and electrical impulses that have evolved over millennia. The experiences with the most potential threat have intensity about them, your emotions are central to remembering them and essential for future predicting. The next time you experience those unconscious fast-acting sensations in your body, you will predict in learnt ways, unconsciously.

## EMOTIONAL HABITS

> Your emotions operate automatically like your thoughts, outside your awareness, locking you into habits that are unhelpful.

The neurological patterns we repeat in our behaviour and our thinking translate into strong networks in our brain. The repeated firing of the neuronal sequence makes that network more efficient. We board these neuronal highways unconsciously and easily – they are our habits. We have many emotional habits.

---

## ACTIVITY 14

Autopilot is a fast, powerful mechanism. If I say, "Twinkle, twinkle little _____"

What happened? You probably said or thought *star* before you even knew it was going to happen. Was it just there automatically without you even trying?

What's your response if I say:

Black and _____

Boys and _____

Night and _____

It's likely that you answered white, girl and day, most people do because you have been acculturated. The world that you live in has taught you the answers, and now they are part of your default patterns, the answers are automatic.

***For you to think of a different answer, you have to slow down and engage some conscious thought, more intentionally using the space between the stimuli and your response.***

Here's another example you might recognise: *how are you?*

Did you automatically say or think: *fine, good, okay, or well thanks*?

All of these are legitimate answers and may sum up how you are perfectly. If you've practised saying "I'm fine" to every inquiry, even when you've been in great distress, you have no doubt developed an automatic pattern, a default network habit. As a result, you may not have developed the skills of emotional literacy, self-care, or those of asking for help. Your emotional wellbeing may be limited by your habitual default pattern of saying you're fine.

Neurologically, you are operating in a problematic loop of cognitive rigidity rather than being psychologically flexible, cognisant, and responsive to the context. You are living unconsciously on autopilot, with rigid thinking that locks you into a narrow range mentally and behaviourally. In this state of autopilot and distraction, emotions remain a mystery and much of the information is outside of your awareness. You are essentially emotionally rigid, hooked on the same repeated thoughts that limit your emotional experience.

## Reflection

- Why would you automatically say "I'm fine" at work, even when you are not? What's the dominant story at play?
- What's the operant emotion/s?
- Is it fear of being seen as weak?
- Is it a need to be seen as perfect, tough, upbeat and resilient?
- Did you miss your own signposts?
- Are you attuned enough to know how your body and mind actually are? If so, are you really fine all of the time?
- Does the habit of saying "I'm fine" serve you well?

Did reading and answering these questions evoke any emotion in you just now?

If it did, sit with it for a minute, what is the signpost telling you?

Next time someone asks you how you are, take a moment to make it an opportunity to grow your emotional intelligence. Check in with your body, be curious to learn how you really feel and see if you can give your state an emotional name beyond fine, good, or okay, even if only to yourself. Over time you will get more comfortable with a wider range of experiences and grow your emotional literacy and accuracy.

## MANAGE YOUR EMOTIONS EFFECTIVELY BY CONSCIOUSLY CHOOSING TO APPROACH OR AVOID

Neurologically speaking, we have two choices to make when it comes to emotions: move away and avoid, or move towards and approach. Both strategies are useful if we use them skilfully.

Avoiding an angry patient is useful and serves your inherent goal to be safe, but avoiding the internal emotional discomfort for its own sake is the enemy of growth and change. In order to develop and progress forward, you will sometimes need to be an amateur, a learner, which can feel vulnerable and uncomfortable. Mastery requires discomfort as you stretch out on your learning edge, expanding your boundaries leaning into the emotional experiences of your life with courage, compassion, and curiosity.

## EMOTIONS EVOKE A SENSE OF VULNERABILITY

Professor Brené Brown is a social researcher and author of several best sellers. Brown studies emotions, particularly courage, vulnerability, shame and empathy. She describes vulnerability as "uncertainty, risk and emotional exposure" and she says that we only get to courage by going through vulnerability.

When you show up to give a patient bad news about their mammogram, to do a procedure while a consultant watches and assesses you, to deliver a baby on your own in a remote location, to fly on retrieval to assist a person who is badly burned, or to sit with a patient whose son has been diagnosed with a learning difficulty, you are vulnerable. Even the act of meeting someone new has a level of vulnerability to it.

> As a doctor, you expose yourself constantly to uncertainty, risk, and emotional vulnerability.

Doctors are raised to consider vulnerability as a weakness, and in many cases decide not to show any vulnerability to their colleagues. Even when we have asked doctors to talk about experiences of kindness, they feel threatened and vulnerable.

In our signature program *Recalibrate*, we invite doctors to reset and tune into their emotions and how they experience them in their bodies. During the program, doctors work in small closed groups of up to 10 people. We ask them to write a story about a time when someone showed them kindness at work. Surprisingly, many doctors find it difficult to start this task. After about five minutes, we ask them to read their stories to their doctor peers in the group. The majority become emotional during this exercise as they read to the group, many of them cry.

We had no idea when we started this group work that noticing kindness would trigger such a response so consistently. What happens? The doctors tell us it is so unfamiliar to tell their stories of receiving kindness that it makes them feel vulnerable. The unfamiliar experience feels risky.

The culture of medicine has encouraged the idea that to be vulnerable is weak and evidence that you cannot handle the work. Plenty of doctors have been told by more senior colleagues that they might not be cut out for the job – a stinging rebuke when you are giving all you have to medicine.

Research into human courage suggests the opposite; vulnerability is a strength. Can you think of someone who has shown courage? Who comes to mind? Did you think of someone who was fearful but proceeded anyway with their intention?

Brown's research has shown that vulnerability is the most accurate measure of courage. She describes being willing to lean in, to be seen even when the outcome is uncertain. This is courage, and it is measured by vulnerability. Harvard Psychologist Susan David researches emotional agility. She says:

"Courage is not the absence of fear but fear walking."

According to Susan David, wanting to avoid vulnerability is wanting dead people's goals. To achieve and strive, to be present, curious, and courageous means taking risks. Connecting with people and being with them in their vulnerability means taking emotional risks.

To be with people who are sick, scared, lost, to be in intimate relationships, to build effective teams, to be loved, and to stretch out to your learning edge all require vulnerability. Staying in your comfort zone limits your opportunity for joy, belonging, and love. If you are not willing to be vulnerable, you are effectively living in fear. To work as a doctor living in fear is not sustainable, fulfilling, or safe.

> Can you choose to live a life that welcomes all emotions skilfully?

In her research, Brown found that the people who were the most resilient embraced vulnerability. They recognised that it was necessary and were willing to do things even when there was no guarantee. She describes them as having a sense of worth and being wholehearted. She says, "Vulnerability is the birthplace of innovation, creativity and change."

To be vulnerable is to be alive – life is not certain. You cannot numb your emotions forever and you cannot selectively numb some emotions. To continue to work your way through medicine flourishing and finding balance and joy, you will need to continue to face fear, anxiety, guilt, shame, and all other emotions.

## I DON'T WANT TO KNOW ABOUT OTHER PEOPLE'S EMOTIONS

You might feel like you want to shy away from this work with emotions because you are worried that the patients will share too much personal information and you won't be able to handle it. Or your colleagues will need too much from you when you feel depleted yourself. What if the patient tells you they feel scared about their operation for instance, or that you let them down somehow? Maybe you won't know how to respond to them. If you brush them off or shut them down, you have missed an opportunity to build trust and confidence. You limit your own perfor-mance, relationships, and wellbeing out of fear.

> **When you can skilfully and accurately understand your own and other's emotions, you are better able to connect, influence, and empathise with them.**

Imagine if you could ramp up your effective connections and com-munications with your patients and colleagues. What would happen? It's likely you would be more responsive and less reactive.

When you can tap into your emotions and the emotions of others, you are connecting on a deeper level. People feel that and trust you more readily. 'People people' are emotionally intelligent, they are using all of the information they have available to connect with others. If you can learn to do this too, you can access more of the information. Patients will confide in you more, telling you things like what they really value and if they intend to follow through with your recommended treatment or not.

## HOW TO RESPOND SPECIFICALLY TO ANXIETY, GUILT AND SHAME

I want to spotlight three emotions that doctors struggle with to help you think about why they arise and to help you frame them in a way that enables you to welcome them as part of your rich full life. Anxiety, guilt, and shame are part of your human experience, they are universal. Like all emotions, they are partly mechanisms of social connection, making sure you stay safe within the tribe. Your social reality will determine how often your brain makes predictions that create these emotions.

Anxiety, guilt, and shame are emotions that can be difficult to hold in your body. You do not need to know everything about why your emotions have arisen in the first place, however, if you experience these emotions as especially sticky, it is important to get some professional help, par-ticularly if your goal is to have more agency and balance in your life. You should not expect to be free of any emotion, but you can learn to work well with them.

Although I will speak to each emotion below, you will notice a clear theme.

1. Breathe.
2. Recognise and name the emotion (take your best guess) – name it to tame it.
3. Sit with it, every emotion is temporary so it will move and shift.
4. Share your experience with a trusted person, practise on the dog or in your journal.
5. Choose your response (accept or take some action).
6. Practise self-compassion.

### Anxiety

Anxiety is a warning signal; it is anticipatory and tells you to be careful. Anxiety is an incredibly useful protector keeping you safe. At the extremes however, anxiety can be immobilising. The best response to anxiety is to lean in; avoidance of whatever is triggering your anxiety usually makes the anxiety worse and leads to other overwhelming emotions like guilt and shame.

You can respond well to anxiety by practising acceptance and by approaching your life with values-based decisions. Acceptance is not apathy; it is a proactive choice about what you do with your energy. You do not control everything in your life. Accept that some things are difficult and unfair. Accept that sometimes you will make mistakes. Accept that you are not perfect, and that perfectionism does not serve you well anyway.

Allow yourself to feel anxiety, as you do... what is important to you. As you lean in with willingness and curiosity you may discover that the sensations of anxiety shift or even subside a little. Approach what causes you anxiety as much as you can, as often as you can. It's okay to avoid your anxiety triggers occasionally when you need a break. Aim for more approach than avoid when it comes to anxiety.

The logic of acceptance is: if there is something you can do, take action and stop worrying. If there is nothing you can do, practise acceptance. Either way, worrying won't help.

If you are anxious about something, ask yourself what is important here, and what you value. For example, you might feel anxious about your exam, but you still want to sit it. Because the exam is of value to you, you feel the anxiety (approach) and do it anyway.

If what you are anxious about is not within your control, practise acceptance. Rumination will not change the course of anything, it will simply deplete your energy. Share your concerns with someone you trust and commit to the ongoing practice of naming anxiety each time it arises.

Avoidance breeds anxiety, with your thoughts amplifying the thing you are worrying about. As you avoid action, your mind makes up stories that may or may not be true in the absence of evidence. You are not testing your thought theories. As much as possible, resist the temptation to stop doing what matters to you.

> Focus on your values, name anxiety, ask for help and lean in.

As you build your approach skills rather than your avoidance skills, you will learn to manage anxiety effectively. Working *with* anxiety rather than getting rid of it is the goal.

**Action Plan:**

Name your anxiety, talk with someone you trust and let them support you as you take committed, values-driven action and design your best life. Accept what you cannot change and lean into what you can.

> Confidence comes with skill and experience, but get some support around you while you build them.

### Guilt

Guilt focuses on your behaviour and tells you that you have done something wrong, motivating you to take reparative action. When you feel guilty, ask yourself *what have I done,* and *is there any repair work I need to do*?

You feel guilt when your values and intentions don't match up with your behaviour. If you have done something wrong, take action, apologise, and reflect on what you can do next time to stay aligned to your values. Guilt is an adaptive emotion; the discomfort of guilt helps us to breach the gap between how we behaved and how we want to be.

> Guilt is a sign of empathy because it has you reviewing how other people feel.

For example, if you are in surgery concentrating on a complex procedure and people keep coming in, asking you how long you will be, pushing to get access to the theatre or asking you questions about other patients, you might eventually lose your patience, telling them loudly and gruffly not to come in again. Later you might feel guilty for the way you spoke, feeling empathy for your colleague who was under pressure from other people. You might find your colleague and apologise to them. Guilt has helped you restore your relationship with your colleague. Remember you are not responsible for their response or their emotions, only your own.

If you are running a version of guilt that is sort of global and you are applying it on a large, generalised scale (something like *"I can't leave medicine because I will disappoint my parents"),* share this with someone you trust, a friend, coach, or psychologist.

Obligation can create guilt. Recognising that you are responsible for the emotional consequences of your choices and taking corrective action will free you from this burden of guilt. Guilt can arise from these kinds of values conflicts: *I want to please my parents and make them proud AND I want to decide my own future.* Be patient, have courage and seek the support you need to take action to create the life you want. Being true to yourself is liberating and mostly admired and respected by others.

There are more options than you think, open up your field of vision and ask yourself what's really possible now that you are an adult out in the world. Be accountable for your emotions, activate your personal agency. Strong emotions like overwhelming guilt can lead to tunnel vision. Our thinking becomes binary which is unhelpful. In this state, we believe either/or is true. Either I am a loyal son, or I am rejecting my family, I cannot be both. More often and/both can be true, it is not necessarily either/or. When you decide to live your own truth, your parents might still also be proud of you. Resist black and white thinking. Open up the field of possibilities to give you some more perspective.

**Action Plan:**

Name guilt to tame it, talk about it with someone you trust and act in service of your own values. Focus on what you need in your life to feel balanced and fulfilled. What matters most to you? Who do you choose to be? In the service of what?

### Shame

Shame is distinguished from guilt by its focus on self rather than behaviour. Shame is an intensely painful experience that has you believing that you are bad and therefore unlovable. Shame threatens your sense of belonging, and so is a difficult psychological challenge that can shape the way you interact with the world because of how you see yourself. When you feel shame, you can feel trapped, powerless and isolated, according to Brown (2006). Guilt says I *did* something bad, shame says I *am* bad. Shame can look and feel like anxiety, but it will not really shift until it is named as shame.

Some evolutionary theorists suggest that shame's role is to make sure people comply with the social norms of the group. Everyone has experienced shame in their life, mostly as a feeling of not being good enough and often expressed as imposter syndrome. It is important to name shame and create some distance – to be able to look at it. Say "shame is here" if you can see it. Most of all, speak it out loud and respond with compassion. Find someone you trust to unravel shame with you.

Unfortunately, shame is incredibly common in medicine. Many

doctors have been humiliated and shamed during their medical training. The culture of competition, perfectionism and 'show no weakness' means that any tiny thing going wrong can be buried inside a doctor as shame. Every day you are at work, you run the risk of something going wrong. If you take that into your *self* as a terrible secret, evidence that you are bad or wrong, you will feel shame. This powerful emotion can then affect the way you predict the world and do untold damage to your relationships.

Shame is highly correlated with addiction, suicide, depression, violence, bullying, eating disorders and aggression. Shame exists in secrecy, silence, and judgement. Shame is felt the same by men and women, but its causes are gendered. According to Brown's research, shame causes women to want to keep up, doing and being everything, and in men it's about never showing any weakness.

Shame centres on your identity, it is a negative self-evaluation that isolates you, inflames your inner critic and affects your ability to show up. A person deep in shame thinks "*I am bad, I am a mistake, I am not good enough*".

> **When you name shame and start talking about it to a trusted person who is empathic, it starts to shift.**

For you to build the life you want and to feel empowered, you need to attend to your shame with compassion. Empathy, self-compassion and support are essential in helping shame move. Brown says, "Shame cannot survive being spoken and being met with empathy." Many doctors have shared their shame with me in coaching and then described the process as having been therapeutic.

**Action Plan:**
Name, shame and understand the vulnerability in it. Respond with self-compassion. As Kristen Neff, author of 'Self Compassion' encourages, talk to yourself as if you are talking to your best friend. Reach out to someone you trust, tell them your story so that together you can keep shame in the daylight, drowning it in empathy.

## SUMMARY

Emotions are a natural part of all our decisions and interactions. Cultivate more positive emotion and stay and be present with the rest, let them be a part of your internal and external communication by working with them rather than wasting energy trying to suppress or ignore them.

Emotions help you connect to others, to understand the external world and your internal world. Whilst it can feel like emotions make you vulnerable, leaning into your emotions can help you learn, connect and progress. The learning that is possible outside your comfort zone is unlimited and, yes, you will be vulnerable sometimes! Working with and processing your emotions is a more effective use of your energy than accumulating emotional baggage.

Emotions are embodied, each with their own physiology. Learning to understand them as signposts that arise out of your brain's predictions can help you be curious, courageous and compassionate towards yourself and others. Improving your emotional literacy improves your self-regulation, your relationships and your day-to-day energy.

Having any given emotion, including anxiety, guilt and shame, is not a problem; knowing how to respond to them is what matters. As you turn toward your emotions, you can experience the rich texture of your life and grow your skills in empathy, compassion and effective communication. Learning when to avoid and when to approach your emotions skilfully gives you a sense of choice in your life, enabling you to respond rather than reacting.

Engaging with your emotions and learning to read them accurately will help you develop your capacity for greater interpersonal skills, empathy and compassion.

### Actions

- Review your own biases and assumptions about the value of emotions.

- Decide to actively improve your emotional literacy by practising using a wider vocabulary to describe your emotions as you experience them. Tune in and share them with others.

- Generate more positive emotions by deciding to include more activities that give you joy. These might include:
  - Spending time with people you care about
  - Doing activities you love
  - Listening to uplifting music
  - Being outside in nature
  - Reflecting on what you are grateful for
  - Exercising
  - Contemplation practice

- Defuse difficult emotions by practising *name it to tame it*. Simply give your emotion a name, allow some space, and practise acceptance in the present moment.

- Instead of "I feel anxious, I feel so guilty", try, "*Anxiety is here, I notice I am experiencing guilt*".

- Start sharing your less intense emotions with someone you trust so that you are practising acknowledging your emotional life, leaning out on your vulnerability edge just a little bit. Talk about emotions with the people around you, recognise their value and own them.

# 7

# COMMUNICATE
# EFFECTIVELY

*"Given the complexity of communication, transformation*
*occurs most readily through small shifts sustained over time."*
— *Oren Jay Sofer*

In this chapter, we will seek to understand the following.

1.  What is effective communication?
2.  The role of empathy and, more importantly, compassion in
    your work.
3.  How to give and receive feedback so that it is useful, not a
    confidence killer.

Communicating effectively with your patients, their families, your
colleagues, and the administrators of your workplace has a huge impact
on how much you enjoy your work. Most often, doctors' training in communication focuses on making patient health outcome and experience
better. The strategies for improved communication in this chapter might
sound familiar as a result, but they are squarely focused on how effective
communication makes a difference for you as the doctor.

This chapter focuses on how you can foster the qualities and skills
of effective communication for your own benefit. We will consider the
role of empathy and compassion in communication, and take a closer
look at how to give and receive feedback so that it can foster insight and
skill development.

At least three of the PERMA elements contributing to flourishing require effective communication; strong supportive relationships, meaningful purpose, and achievement. However, since positive emotions and engagement emanate from the other three elements, we might argue that all of the elements of flourishing require effective communication.

Doctors are assumed to have effective communication skills more than is the reality. Medicine typically has not used systems and processes like performance review, customer service training, or worker wellbeing to help promote great communication in the same way other industries have. Funding models, time pressure and a preponderance to science has given priority to task achievement rather than the skills of interpersonal connection. Your ability to communicate well is assumed, partly because of your intelligence and high level of education, rightly or wrongly.

Managing and developing the performance of doctors is non-existent in most healthcare organisations. Relationship skills and leadership training has rarely been offered to doctors, and healthcare systems have been oblivious to fostering provider wellbeing until very recently. Feedback is not given (or given poorly) and bullying and harassment has been rife. Junior doctors have had no voice. One way or another, many doctors have felt completely disempowered, unable to communicate their needs or to advocate on their own behalf.

Unconscious bias and assumption are often at the root of miscommunication. If you have endeavoured to make a complaint, create a boundary or address a systems problem like workflow or roster, you may have been labelled a difficult or disruptive doctor. If you are female, you may have been labelled emotional or much worse by others in the system. If you were born in another country or are a person of colour, you may continue to be undermined, no matter how much experience you have. These experiences and labels can be hard to shake, reducing your influence and, more importantly, your confidence.

Your communication skills could make or break your medical career. So how do you learn the skills for effective communication and how do you know when you are successfully implementing what you have learnt?

> Doctors develop their communication skills in laissez-faire ways,
> systems for feedback are poorly executed and actively avoided.

Imagine an alternative universe to the one you work in now, where you consistently communicate well with everyone – patients, their families, your colleagues, the administrators of the hospital, the health department bureaucrats. Imagine they also communicate effectively. You can say what you mean and so can they without confusion or conflict. Relationships are high in trust and respect; you feel psychologically safe. Your mental and emotional energy is available for clear thinking, curiosity, creativity, compassion, and connection.

Imagining a better way is a useful tool for establishing what you need so that you can create a better option. While this utopia might sound like a fantasy, you can create pockets of this in your life with the right skills once you know what you're aiming for.

> When you are an effective communicator, your relationships are
> smoother, people trust you, and there is less conflict in your life. This
> has a direct impact on your energy, mood, and confidence, giving you
> more opportunity to flourish.

## WHAT IS EFFECTIVE COMMUNICATION?

The purpose of communication is to connect and build understanding through shared information and stories – giving and receiving information verbally, in writing, and otherwise, so that we can understand ourselves, others, and the world. Communication is how we make things happen in our lives. It's the catch all word that describes activities designed to share our thoughts, perceptions, emotions, and experiences. Sometimes communication is as much about what we don't say as what we do say.

> Most importantly, communication is how we connect and bond, or don't!

Every gesture of communication we make to others has been generated by an internal experience – a belief, a habit, a choice. That's why the work you have done in earlier chapters on your internal environment is important for how effectively you communicate with others. Your internal dialogue is communicated to yourself and to others through words and stories, voice pitch and tone, facial expressions, body postures, silences. Much of what you communicate is outside of your awareness.

Messages can be conscious or unconscious and be sent with or without words. Many messages are implied. Sometimes other people are receiving messages from you that you don't even realise you are sending, subconsciously folding your arms, for instance. As meaning-making creatures, we interpret and predict the world from our unique reality. We describe this reality to ourselves inside our own heads and to others, through story.

Your *intention* is central to effective communication. **It's effective when the intention is activated and understood by others** – the message is clear, concise, coherent, and understood. The person sending the message is able to say what they mean, and the receiver is able to *interpret it accurately*. Agreement is not what makes it *effective*. Nor is an absence of emotion indicative of effective communication.

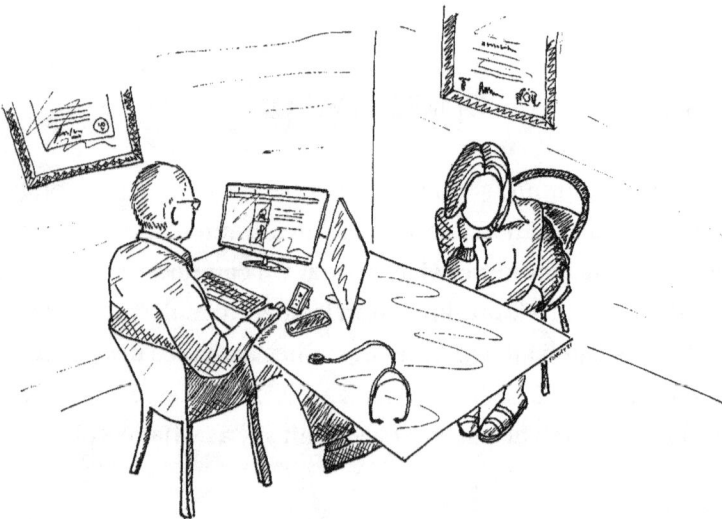

I am your patient and tell you that I have felt nauseous and feverish for the past 24 hours, and I've also been vomiting. I want you to understand my experience so that you can help me. I hope that you will connect enough with my story that you will want to help me. I am communicating the technical details, my symptoms, and my human experience. My story includes my emotions. What you hear, feel, and think about what I share with you is not in my control and is determined by your cognitive templates which create your unique reality.

If you look distracted – looking at your computer or your watch – I might receive the implied message that you are not really listening, that you don't care, or that you don't know what to do. My guesses could be true, or not. You might care deeply but be distracted by your own internal voice that is worrying about the previous patient.

We each interpret messages within our own context. The effectiveness of our communication is contingent on testing or checking our interpretations with each other. As I apologise for taking too much of your time, you realise that you are communicating disinterest or distraction with your body and turn to face me, communicating that your interest and attention are now on what I am saying.

> **Our communication is only truly effective when the intended message is the one that is received.**

## CARE IS WHAT MAKES COMMUNICATION EFFECTIVE

Communication is a two-way street; it relies on both the sender and the receiver of the messages. Understanding each other only happens well when we care about *what* is being shared, or we care about the person *who* is sharing. Notice it's caring that's important; we don't have to agree.

Effective communication is not only about sending messages, it also involves our capacity to receive messages. If your outbound messages are not received in the way you intended, it is up to you to adapt and send the message again in a new way. When you receive a message, it is also up to you to confirm if you have received the message in the way it was intended.

The more invested the parties are in the shared act of communicating, the higher chance there is of improving the communication, even if it provokes intense emotion or is challenging to resolve. This is why investing in strong personal relationships high in respect and trust makes a difference to your experience of work. Even if people don't care about the content, they still care about each other and that makes a difference to how they behave.

> **At the base of effective communication is care.**

## Lincoln's Story

*Lincoln is the medical director in a large regional hospital and has just had an argument with Tom, who is the administrator responsible for workforce. Tom is highly stressed about his budget and the number of locum doctors he needs to employ to keep the emergency department and the on-call roster staffed. In turn, Lincoln is frustrated by the lack of senior doctors working in the ED. He is concerned for the safety of the patients and the junior doctors, saying they will need to close the ED overnight some nights due to the lack of senior doctors available. Unfortunately, what he doesn't know is that the CEO has already told Tom that shutting the ED is not an option. Tom and Lincoln end up shouting at each other. The situation seems impossible; they both feel like there is no way out.*

*Lincoln feels fed up, but he takes some time to think about a new way to tackle the communication. He tells himself that regardless of his frustrations, he wants his community to be safe. The reputation of the hospital and the safety of staff and patients are important to him. Lincoln also cares about resolving this issue so that his own stress can go down – at the moment he is thinking about the risks constantly. Even though the very thought of re-opening the conversation is anxiety provoking, given the terse interaction they have just had, Lincoln decides to ask Tom if he will agree to a meeting with him and the CEO.*

*Tom agrees to the meeting. He cares about this too.*

They both care deeply, which is why the issue is 'hot' for them both and why they each decide it is worth the effort to meet again, even though it's very uncomfortable. Each person makes a values-based decision guided by what matters to them. The reality remains: the problem is complex, the communication is difficult, and their emotions are intense.

To send and receive messages that result in understanding and connection, we need to care. If you don't care, it doesn't really matter if others understand or what the outcomes are. If you don't really care, there is no point communicating. You may as well talk to a brick wall.

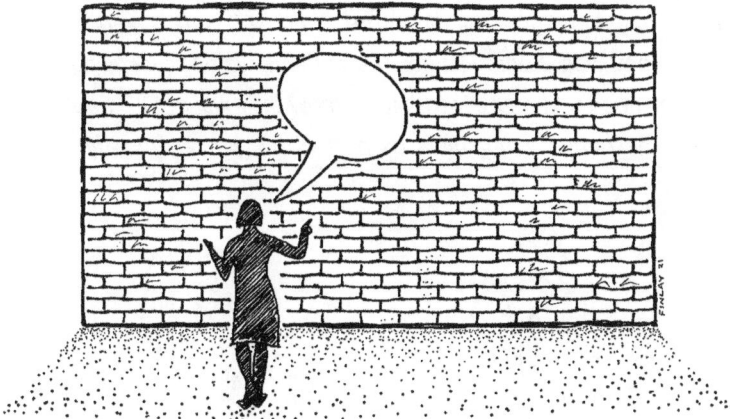

This is also the problem with the many cc emails you receive. How many do you open and read with curiosity? Why is it that you don't open these emails? You probably answered these questions with something like *I don't need to know, they're not interested in my opinion anyway,* or *I don't care.* If you said *you don't have enough time,* that is really code for *the email is not a priority.* In other words, *I don't care enough to open it,* or *I have more important things I give my energy to or care about.*

Still, the message can get complicated because the receiver of the message may wonder why you don't care. Of course, you may care a great deal but be unwell in bed or out of the country, or you may not have even received the message in the first place if it was sent electronically. Checking and clarifying are markers of effective communication. Assumptions and bias, as we have seen, hinder effective communication.

> As the sender and the receiver, it pays to be curious, to follow up, to ask questions, and to avoid assumption.

# Reem's Story

*Reem works as a GP in a busy suburban clinic. Her stress response has been activated all morning because she's been running late from the very first patient of the day. All the patients since have told her how frustrated they are to have sat in her waiting room for a long time. She cares deeply about this, which is why she feels so stressed. But she cares more about the patient in front of her getting her full attention and good medical care. The result is that every patient pays in time as they wait. Reem justifies the patients waiting by saying to herself, "When they need a longer consult, they know they will get it". Reem is willing to accept the patient complaints as part of the process for the good care she provides.*

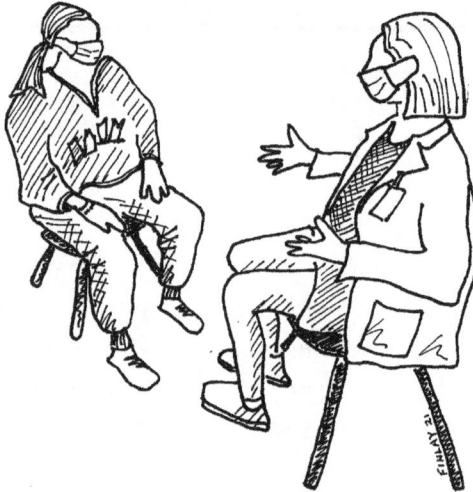

Reem is prioritising – she cares more about having enough time with the patients than about people waiting. The patients who know this will happen every time they come to see Reem and continue to book with her are implicitly saying they are willing to wait. That does not necessarily mean they are happy. They may decide they have no other choice because there is no other doctor available, or perhaps they prefer to wait in Reem's waiting room more than in the emergency department at the hospital. Context is always relevant to our decisions and our emotional state.

Communication that is more effective would include timely advice to patients about what's happening. For instance, patients could be encouraged to phone the clinic before their appointment to ask if Reem is on time. Or perhaps an online tracking system could be implemented that allows patients to see from home what the estimated wait time will be in the hours before their appointment with Reem.

> Understanding, care, and connection are the hallmarks of effective communication and context is important.

## HOW TO START LEARNING ABOUT YOUR COMMUNICATION HABITS

### ACTIVITY 15

### My communication habits

**Try this**

Think of the most tedious person you know. What happens inside you when they start talking?

Now think of the most captivating conversation you have had recently. What caught your attention and held it? What happened inside of you?

Is your communication different when you care more? In what ways?

To learn more about communication, you need to explore your own reactions to your real-life communication. As you notice what works and doesn't work for you, make a commitment to adjust *how* you communicate. Don't leave it to autopilot if you truly want to raise your effectiveness.

## Reflection

You can ask yourself these questions as the speaker or the listener to find out more about yourself as a communicator. You can ask them internally in real time or as a reflective practice in hindsight. Either way, make a conscious decision to use what you observe to guide you towards becoming a more effective communicator.

1.   Does this communication matter to me?
2.   Does the topic matter to me?
3.   Does the other person matter to me?
4.   Does our relationship matter to me?
5.   Is it more important to be accurate or connected in this moment?

The same questions apply to your inner dialogue. When you are ruminating, stuck, or feeling emotional about something in your life, ask yourself:

1.   Do I really care about this topic, does it hold any meaning for me?
2.   What is it specifically that matters to me?
3.   Now consciously choose what you want to do. Use your energy and attention wisely. Does it matter?

     Yes: pay attention and decide what action is needed. If there is no action to take, practise acceptance.

     No: can you park it? Practise acceptance and put your energy into something you do care about.

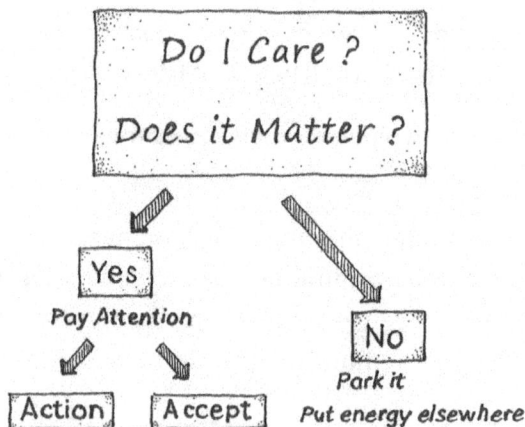

Do I Care ?
Does it Matter ?

Yes
Pay Attention

Action   Accept

No
Park it
Put energy elsewhere

Your answers to these questions are contextual. You may have different responses on different days, that's to be expected and is normal. For example, if your partner is telling you about their day at work when you are trying to go to sleep after your own exhausting day, you might not care very much in that moment. If they are telling you over dinner, you might be totally absorbed in what they are sharing.

Asking yourself what matters means guiding your participation in communication with your values. As you go to sleep, rest might have more value in that moment than listening to your partner. As you listen over dinner, your relationship with your partner might be the only value you care about. If your partner says in the middle of the night, *I'm taking our son to the hospital*, this communication will probably matter enormously whatever you are doing, including if you are in a deep sleep.

Sometimes it is the content, sometimes it is the relationship or the person that matters. Either way, these simple questions can help you respond more effectively to your inner dialogue and to other people. You can also invite other people to ask you these questions as a means of learning about your own communication habits. There is no one script to roll out every time because context always matters.

## SO WHY IS EFFECTIVE COMMUNICATION IMPORTANT IN MEDICINE?

### *Patients and their families*

Every person using the health system as a patient has a problem they are seeking to change or fix. Even if the patient is simply seeking your reassurance, they are vulnerable by virtue of being the patient. Your role as doctor is to help them. As you know, you are not always as able to help them as they hope.

Every interaction with a patient includes emotion. You hold the balance of power because of your role and your knowledge – of anatomy, the specific problem, possible treatments, and the health system. Your ability to understand their story and the problem, to share information, respond constructively to the patient's questions and emotions, and to guide them through the relevant processes are all contingent on your communication skills, which are contingent in any moment on your state.

When things go badly, part of your role as doctor is to be able to deliver accurate information and respond to your patients and their families' reactions. Your capacity to communicate effectively in these difficult contexts of other people's intense emotion and confusion is a part of the medical and therapeutic treatment you offer your patients and their support people. If you are not able to do so, you run the risk of doing harm to them.

This is an incredibly high bar, one that you as a doctor are measured against every day – one that you likely expect of yourself too, even when you are depleted. How you communicate and how you respond internally to all of this will affect where you are on the wellbeing continuum, and it is highly dynamic.

### Colleagues

Medical care is delivered to patients by teams of people and in silos. Both systems of delivery require you to communicate with your colleagues if the patient is to receive the best possible care. Ego, hierarchy, and pressure can interfere with effective communication in teams.

Medicine trains doctors using an apprentice model, meaning there is a clear pecking order. More experienced doctors showed you how to do your work; show one, do one, teach one. While you shadowed other doctors on ward rounds and sat as a student watching other doctors communicating with patients and other health professionals, you probably learnt what *not* to do as much as what to do. If you were lucky, some of these more senior doctors might have reflected with you about what you witnessed and helped you crystallise the micro skills of great communication.

You might be involved in committees or on research teams. These require effective communication skills if you are to advance what you care about. To build your influence and make an impact in the areas you care about, you need to be able to use your voice, maintain your focus in the face of challenge, tolerate uncertainty, be politically savvy, and connect with others to advance your work.

You don't have to like everyone or agree with everyone. You do want to be able to connect, share your ideas, and influence the world you work in, so the more people you can communicate effectively with, the more empowered you can be and the more you can advance what gives your life meaning. A life filled with meaning and a capacity to act with purpose achieving your goals is satisfying and builds momentum and positive energy. This is what a thriving doctor looks and sounds like. They are able to meet their psychological needs of survival, belonging, and autonomy. They have the five elements of PERMA active in their life.

> **You can make a positive difference in the world for yourself and for others when you communicate with accuracy, care and connection.**

## HOW TO COMMUNICATE EFFECTIVELY

### ACTIVITY 16

### A doctor role-model communicator

Call to mind a doctor you know who is the most effective communicator you've seen in action (if you can't think of a doctor, think of the most effective communicator you know).

- What are the key **qualities** they model?
- What **attitudes** do they seem to live by?
- What **behaviours** do they exhibit that let you know they are effective in their communication?

What qualities, attitudes and behaviours did you notice in the effective communicator doctor you thought of? Write them down and reflect if *you* use these qualities, attitudes, and behaviours in your communication.

Do you give priority to the same things? Where does your attention and energy go when you communicate with others?

Did you notice the quality of presence in the person you thought of? Have you ever been in conversation with someone and felt like you were the only person in the room, as though what you had to say was the most important insight known to mankind?

They were totally present to you, and you felt like they cared about you.

> **Great communicators are present.**

Maybe when you thought of the most effective doctor communicator you've met, you noticed how they interacted with an attitude of open curiosity. They seem eager to learn or understand. Perhaps they seemed to genuinely seek the truth or were willing to rethink their own position. Perhaps you noticed that they were open to possibilities, they hadn't already made up their mind or only sought to confirm their existing view (cognitive rigidity).

Effective communicators seek first to understand, they listen with curiosity and an intent to learn. They deeply value a new perspective, a challenge to their own potential cognitive rigidity. You might have noticed how they rarely interrupt, how they ask others what they think before sharing their own view, or how they listen with kindness. These skills build trust and a sense of safety. They are ready to change their mind and say they made a mistake if that becomes apparent, because they care about the relationship and learning.

> **Effective communicators are fully present and listen deeply with intent and curiosity, seeking first to understand. This attitude builds trust and safety.**

# THE QUALITIES OF GREAT COMMUNICATION

## *Be Present*

If you are thinking about something else when someone is talking to you then you are not listening carefully, and you are not observing the non-verbal cues available. If your patient is describing their pain or asking you a technical question about their surgery but you are thinking about the next patient, you are not communicating *effectively*, even if you think you look like it.

> **The key quality of effective communication is presence.**

There are many distractions in the medical environment which invite you to multitask. Our brains are not actually capable of complex multi-tasking, only simple things like walking and talking about well-known or habituated topics. To be truly innovative in our problem solving and to listen deeply to understand another person's experience, we need to be single focused. If you want to communicate *effectively* with someone else, you need to give them your full attention.

Be present to whomever you are with and to whatever is happening inside your own mind and body. Practising mindfulness will strengthen your skills in presence.

> **Single tasking will improve your capacity to communicate effectively.**

Research into multitasking is very clear: we make more errors, feel more stressed and waste more time when we multitask. Multitasking, more accurately named switch tasking, is inefficient and ineffective. It causes our brains to use more oxygen and more glucose as it switches in and out of neurological pathways and networks.

Although it feels counterintuitive, slowing down will help you speed up. Find one or two areas of your work that you can single task and practise often. Finish one task at a time and observe with an open mind. Don't start with the most complex part of your work, some systems force you to multitask. If you are reading results or a report, practise being fully present on that one task whenever you can, even if it only amounts to 10 minutes a day. Notice if you are more efficient, make less errors and feel less stressed.

> **Presence changes everything about communication.**

### Be Curious

Seek first to understand. Effective communicators have an attitude of curiosity and openness – it is not all about them telling and knowing. As the curious message sender, you remain interested in understanding the other person's needs and values and learning about their experiences and what they care about.

As a doctor, you might feel worried that all this seeking to understand and active caring will take up too much time in the practical sense, and too much energy in the emotional sense. A Harvard study found that 56% of doctors believed they did not have time to show patients compassion. Researchers from John Hopkins University wanted to find out. In a randomised controlled trial, they found that it took doctors 40 seconds to show enough compassion to cancer patients to reduce their anxiety significantly. Their study has been replicated with similar results. In an average of 40 seconds, doctors were able to reduce their patients' anxiety significantly, making a meaningful difference to their wellbeing.

Patients in the enhanced compassion intervention rated their oncologist more caring, sensitive, compassionate, and warm. The patients' perception of their doctor made a difference to their health. It turns out caring, connecting, and communicating effectively with a patient can take less than a minute and is *treatment* too.

Anaesthetist Robin Youngson also sought to understand this concern often cited by doctors that caring takes too long. He wrote about it in his book '*A Time to Care*', concluding that when a doctor takes a little time to listen to a patient and understand them, they build a kind of trust that makes their work together much more efficient in the longer term because they are able to get to the important information quicker.

Many medical writers and researchers (Halpin, Trzeciak and Mazzarelli, Epstein) have concluded that there are very few outlier patients and colleagues who talk too much and too long. This fear just doesn't seem to materialise. It's a story doctors tell themselves. A little bit of curiosity at the beginning of a relationship goes a long way in medical care. Perhaps this is a story you would like to challenge in your work, if this is interesting to you, run some experiments.

## Mark's Story

*Mark works as a cardiologist staff specialist in a large metropolitan hospital. The department is understaffed, and he is busy all the time. There have been many times when there is no one else to see patients, and he feels the pressure. He is conscious of working with people who have had cardiovascular events and the link generally with stress. Recent research has endorsed mindfulness practices for people with cardiovascular disease. Mark has been trying to role model mindfulness to his patients by taking a little more time with them.*

*Initially, he was very agitated that his experiment was showing him to be naïve and unrealistic! However, after the first anxiety provoking month, he told me that it was now taking him about the same time to see his patients – he goes home from work at the same time as he used to. He said it wasn't what he was doing that was so different, more how he was doing it. Mark said that the main difference to come out of his experiment was that he feels much less stressed. He is no longer agitated about the time and has a feeling of space in his day.*

*Mark began his experiment because he thought it would be good for his patients, and he discovered that it's also good for him. His experiment continues. He is more curious than ever to observe what happens for the patients and himself now that he has let go of the 'I haven't got time' story.*

### Reflection

- Can you think of a time when you have been curious and connected to what another person was communicating?
- What happened inside of you? What happened externally in your behaviour?
- Did you feel more free to share your thoughts and feelings? Did you ask more questions? Did you learn more or feel more valued?
- Did this kind of interaction feel more satisfying?
- Did you feel more engaged?

> Curiosity is the foundation of learning. When you are communicating with curiosity, you make different kinds of connections with people and with information.

## *Be Kind*

### How to Listen and Observe Deeply

Kindness is powerful because it is discretionary. You can do much of your job without being kind. When you do it with kindness, the other person feels it and knows that you made an active choice purely because you could. Think about the last time one of your colleagues was kind to you at work. Perhaps they stopped to help you when they were under pressure; maybe they offered to cover for you so you could get home; maybe they apologised for some minor incursion earlier in the day. Kindness is a synonym for compassion.

Kindness creates positive emotion (the first PERMA factor) and is contagious. An intention to communicate with kindness primes you and those you are communicating with to connect and care. Kindness in this context boosts the immune system, increases the production of oxytocin, and can reduce blood pressure.

> Kindness builds trust, creating a sense of belonging and safety and inviting vulnerability. Kindness encourages better communication, more care and more connection.

You can show that you care about other people by being present with them and curious about their experience. As a doctor, one of the fastest and most effective ways you can show you care is to listen with kindness.

Researchers in 2018 found that seven out of ten doctors interrupted their patients with a median time of 11 seconds – just a couple of sentences into their story. Patients who were allowed to talk freely took between two and 108 seconds. Doctors who consistently interrupt like this have a habit they are probably not even aware of. What unconscious assumptions do you think the doctor has that leads to them so readily interrupting the person they are caring for?

The most precious currency for the doctors I work with is time. Like the doctors in the Harvard study, most don't believe they have enough time, and many say one of their developmental goals is to improve their time management.

Trzeciak and Mazzarelli write in their book '*Compassionomics*' about a myriad of research demonstrating that perception of not having enough time might unnecessarily and negatively affect patient care. The research shows that spending an extra minute connecting compassionately with your patient can alter your perception of time. In essence, slowing down to help someone else creates a perception of more time. This is what the researchers call time affluence. They suggest that helping someone elevates our sense of purpose and efficacy and these positive emotions change our perception of time.

Trzeciak and Mazzarelli conclude that helping others a little more slowly with conscious, compassionate intent makes a difference to how you perceive time. The positive effect of this process activates your reward pathways in your brain, buffering the stress pathways and at least temporarily helping you forget your own worries. Trzeciak describes his own burnout experience, saying he believes after reviewing the compassion research that it can be the antidote to burnout for caregivers, including doctors.

> When you meet your patients and colleagues with presence, curiosity, and kindness, they trust you. This has a positive impact on both of you.

## SKILLS FOR EFFECTIVE COMMUNICATION

The pace and the complexity of medicine interferes with effective communication. When you are under pressure and stressed, you narrow your attention, including your listening. You are more likely to interrupt, less likely to be creative in your problem solving, less aware of your environment, and more likely to miss information.

To communicate effectively, you need to ensure that those you're communicating with receive your messages in the way you intended them. You need to be able to seek clarity about whether you have understood the messages they are sending you. This cycle of sending, receiving and clarifying is continuous and recognises that individual difference plays a role in interpreting messages that can make communication ineffective.

Three key skills for effective communication are:

1. Listening with your whole body
2. Maintaining awareness
3. Building trust.

### Listen with your whole body

Notice where your feet are facing – are they pointing at the door? Notice if your arms are crossed over your body, creating a barrier. Are you aware of the messages you are sending? Practising mindfulness raises your awareness to these behaviours and helps you pay attention to what you need to change in the way you communicate.

Facing the other person, smiling at them, nodding for them to keep going, and making appropriate eye contact and encouraging sounds all help the other person know that you are listening and you care. There are many structural things that can interfere with your communication: masks, goggles, machinery, computers, other people. These factors can cause distraction and disconnect. Use your body to communicate your intention. Demonstrate your presence, curiosity, and kindness physically.

Listen for emotions, notice what isn't said, and test your accuracy by reframing and checking received information with the sender as a way of asking if you've understood them.

As Maya Angelou wisely observed, people will forget what you said and did, "...But they will never forget how you made them feel". Your ability to make other people feel seen and heard is a powerful unconscious and conscious connection skill.

> When people feel seen and heard by you, rapport and trust are established easily.

You can amplify your communication skills by      also      listening carefully to your own body when you are listening to another person. Your body is constantly giving you messages about your safety. Your own physiology shifts when you are in a safe or unsafe situation. You are unlikely to be truly curious and linger in a communication if you feel unsafe. Staying attuned to how your body is showing up in the communication gives you the opportunity to respond rather than react on autopilot. When you are mindfully present to your own body, you can keep adjusting and improving your communication. These tiny real-time adjustments enhance your effectiveness and allow you to use your emotional intelligence.

As we know, doctors regularly interrupt their patients within a few seconds consultation. Research by social psychologists has found that doctors interrupt patients they don't like more often, and that people with more power in organisations interrupt more in meetings. It is up to you to practise your listening skills if you want to be more effective in your communication.

Make a commitment to improving your listening skills by actively practising in small bursts. You might like to start practising at home, or with your reception staff, or your first two patients every day. As you start to feel a little more natural and comfortable in your listening, stretch out, practise for the first hour of the day, and practise not interrupting someone you know you always interrupt.

In meetings, practise waiting before you speak. Let others share their ideas first, especially if you are the chair or the most powerful person in the room. If others say what you think then don't speak at all. Learn to be a listener as much as you are a talker. You might learn some things, after all you already know what *you* know. If you do all the talking, you limit the time there is for learning. Take a long slow breath and use your body to be present and available to listen deeply. Remember you have two ears and one mouth and aim to make that your ratio guide for a while as you learn the skill of deep listening.

Improving your listening skills so that you can be an effective communicator takes real-time practice, it is not something you can learn in theory. Very effective communicators are the people who can maintain their care and connection even under pressure, and they can do it well because they are practising all the time.

> **Effective communication is not about demonstrating how much you know, it's about enhancing the collective understanding and progressing forward with good will.**

## Reflection

- Is it more important for you to show how much you know or to learn something new?
- Is it more important to be the smartest person in the room or to be the most connected person in the room?
- What is your intention when you communicate? What message do you want the others to receive?
- What is your intention as the listener?

### *Awareness - Your Reality Is Not My Reality*

Effective communication involves words, body language, tone, pitch, facial expression, and the unsaid. You are constantly unconsciously sifting and sorting information, deciding what to ignore, what to focus on, and what's missing. As you know from earlier chapters, our brain is a predicting machine that uses past experiences, established neuronal pathways, and an assessment of the safety of the environment to decipher what is going on in the world. This means that each receiver of information is unique with their own biases and assumptions built into their predictions.

> When emotion is involved, you notice non-verbal cues more than you notice words. You mostly receive these messages unconsciously.

## Gina's Story

*Gina has started working in a new hospital. This is her third week. She approaches Martin as he is finishing up. Martin has worked at the hospital for six years and is responsible for the rostering. Gina asks Martin a question about a shift in a month's time that she'd like to swap with someone. She is polite and warm in her approach.*

*Martin has been on call the last two nights and has been at the hospital most of the time. He has been fielding rostering questions constantly for the past few days. He believes a doctor should coordinate the roster because an admin person doesn't understand all the implications, but after doing it for two years he's starting to think someone else should take a turn. He brushes Gina off, telling her he's on his way home and she should send him an email. Martin doesn't look her in the eye, and although she notices he looks tired, she thinks to herself, "He didn't need to be so rude".*

*Gina wonders if she is going to be okay at this hospital; it was such a struggle last year at her previous job.*

If you are depleted or under pressure, a seemingly straightforward question can easily become a very ineffective exchange or even a conflict.

When we are depleted, it is much harder to regulate our emotions and our thinking. This is amplified if both parties are depleted. Moments like these happen thousands of times a day in medicine.

It's worth remembering HALLTSS when it comes to communication – if you are hungry, angry, late, lonely, tired, stressed or sick, your communication will be negatively affected. You cannot control the high pressure, complex environment of medical work. The skills of self-awareness (stress management, emotional intelligence, effective self-regulation) will help you to manage your communication more effectively.

> **Your capacity to remain aware, well regulated, less stressed, and emotionally attuned will help you be an effective communicator in the moment, not just in hindsight.**

Of course, your humanness means you will get it wrong sometimes, none of us are our best selves under pressure. It is part of the human condition to be *less* than you planned some of the time. If you are depleted because you have been on call, recognise that this will have a detrimental impact on your abilities. Learn what those impacts are and take action to meet them. Remember you are human, go for excellence or even 'good enough' when you are under pressure, perfection is a myth. You can do a quick assessment of what happens to you under pressure or stress by answering these five questions.

### Reflection

When you are under pressure or stressed:

- Do you become more task focused (abrupt, instructional, directive, authoritative)?
- Do you tune out and lose your concentration?
- Do you forget things and fail to pay attention to details?
- Are you more reactive and more likely to be short tempered?
- Are you distracted and vague?

If you are not sure what happens to your communication under pressure, go back to the questions in Activity 15, earlier in this chapter. If there is someone you work with and trust, perhaps you can ask them what they've noticed. Think back to the doctor you recalled earlier who is an effective communicator (Activity 16), and watch them with the intent to learn. If you can't think of a doctor who is an effective communicator, look outside medicine for role models. Find yourself a trusted buddy, mentor, or coach who you can seek feedback from.

### Build Trust

Our brain's mirror neurons and the hormone oxytocin are the bonding structures of our body that help us connect and respond positively to each other. When we feel seen and heard, these systems in our body activate us to take more risks, share more, be more vulnerable, speak up and ask questions, challenge the status quo, and share what matters most.

George's Story

*George is an anaesthetist. His patient, Samira, shared a past trauma with him because she was wondering if that's what was making her anxious about her surgery. George stayed with her and listened for another minute or two, allowing her to say out loud what was worrying her. This reassured her, and she seemed to calm a little. George couldn't control Samira's response, but his relaxed manner and willingness to listen without discounting her experience made a difference. This in turn had a positive impact on the whole surgical team. This interaction took George a little longer at the beginning, but ultimately made the whole interaction smoother and easier, overall saving time and energy for the healthcare team and Samira.*

Those two minutes of effective communication can alter the way both people go on to predict the world and the emotions they generate. Day after day, this can add up to more ease and joy in your work.

> Communication is more effective with presence, curiosity, kindness,
> trust, and care. You might recognise the qualities of mindfulness
> in effective communication.

## DOES EMPATHY MAKE COMMUNICATION EFFECTIVE?

Empathy is critical to good doctoring according to medical schools around the world. Yet research has shown that medical students' empathy for their patients declines from the third year of their studies. What happens?

Many of the doctors I work with who are preparing for clinical exams tell me in our practice sessions that they will be empathic towards the patient. When I ask them what that means and how they will demonstrate it in their presentation or role play with the actor patient, a good number of them don't know.

What do you think it means to be empathic?

What are the behaviours of empathy?

Empathy is the key skill in seeking to understand another person's experience. Empathy is actively seeking to understand what life is like for another person, through their lens and context, not your own. If you do not understand yourself first and know your own values, it is incredibly difficult to listen and perceive the world from someone else's view, because your own unconscious biases and assumptions get in the way. In empathy, you seek to see the world through another person's biases and predictions. Oren Jay Sofer is a teacher of nonviolent communication. In his book '*Say What You Mean,*' he describes empathy as "An endeavour to inhabit both an emotional and an embodied understanding of another's experience". The kind of empathy doctors describe trying to develop to me is more cognitive empathy. True empathy invites us to "Reach for our shared humanity" (Sofer 2018 p 103).

> To be empathic, we need to understand by listening
> patiently with curiosity.

## Reflection

- Who's the most empathic person you know?
- How can you tell they are empathic?
- How do you *feel* when they empathise with you?
- How do you feel when someone else sees the world as you do?

> Being seen and heard, trusted and valued, is the ideal environment for growing, learning, and connecting.

Many doctors who have written about becoming a patient have said that it caused them to be a different doctor – a better doctor. The late Dr Chris O'Brien, head and neck surgeon at Sydney's RPA, is one example. Unfortunately, Chris died of brain cancer in 2009. Seeing the world as a patient altered Chris's view, he felt more empathy for his patients. As a result, he spoke publicly about different elements of his journey, for instance, the value of his newfound meditation practice for his own well-being. Lived experience is a powerful teacher, but we don't need to go to such lengths to improve our capacity for empathy.

> Meeting your patients with the qualities and intentions already described will raise your empathy as you connect with others because you care.

But can caring too much damage your own wellbeing? Many doctors worry that the emotional burden will be too much. Emotional empathy can create a great deal of pain in the person experiencing the empathy.

Some researchers have found that doctors higher on empathy scales have more satisfaction in their work and less burnout. However, there is contradictory research that suggests that empathy leads to emotional overload and fatigue.

> Neurologically, when you are empathising with another person's pain,
> your own pain network is activated.

The same neurons that activate when you are in pain are active as you empathise with another, especially if you unconsciously recognise them as like you or part of your *in group.* In the extreme, it can become impossible for you to distinguish what is your pain and what is the other person's pain. This is the very real burden of emotional labour that becomes emotional fatigue. Pure empathy is not a sustainable practice for you when your work has you meeting people every day who are in pain. Empathy on its own can feel like endless suffering. It doesn't take too long before you feel buried in pain. Of course, you want to prevent that from happening.

Some researchers and social psychologists say cognitive empathy is the answer. This kind of empathy is more detached. Cognitive empathy means you seek to take the other person's perspective as a thinking exercise, as a means of understanding what is happening for them. Psychiatrist and philosopher Dr Jodi Halpern has studied these issues for decades. She says in her book, '*From Detached Concern to Empathy*', that doctors who are practising detached concern are not more rational and are less likely to notice medical errors. She says, "Skilful empathy elevates [medical] work contributing to the meaningfulness of people's lives". She concludes that empathy builds a therapeutic alliance that improves medical effectiveness.

Neurological research has found that empathy and compassion activate different networks in the brain, and that activating compassion may have benefits in terms of sustained carer wellbeing. Perhaps this is the way to resolve the friction between wanting to be empathically attuned to others and not overwhelmed.

## COMPASSION MAKES A MEDICAL LIFE MORE SUSTAINABLE THAN EMPATHY ALONE

In compassion, your neurological reward network is activated. The dopamine involved in your reward system helps you feel good and activates your desire to want to take action to help relieve the other person's suffering. This is the fundamental difference between empathy and compassion.

> With empathy you seek to understand and resonate with the human experience of the person you are with. With compassion you seek to relieve their suffering.

It is the *active* element of compassion that distinguishes it from empathy.

> You can think of compassion as empathy + action.

In both scenarios, you look empathic as you stay with the other person's emotions and story, listening with presence, curiosity and kindness and building trust and connection. If I were observing you, I may not notice any difference in your behaviour.

> The difference between empathy and compassion is in your internal dialogue, your intention, and your neuronal network.

Internally, you are aware of wanting to relieve the person's suffering. In compassion, your self-talk is recognising that being with the person, listening deeply and honouring their experience is of value and has the potential to relieve their suffering. Understanding and feeling the other person's pain is not enough. Listening with empathy, your internal dialogue may discount what is happening. You may say something like, *'Well I couldn't do much, all I did was listen to them.'*

> Neurologically, compassion fatigue is a misnomer. This experience of feeling overwhelmed by other's pain is more accurately named empathy fatigue.

Empathy is an important part of compassion. It is not useful to make it the bad guy, it is simply not enough on its own. Practising compassion by extending empathy to include action is a more sustainable way for you to practise medicine. Feeling your common humanity and recognising it as valuable is sustaining for you in the moment and over time.

> You can change your patient's experience of healthcare by being empathic. You can improve both of your experiences by being compassionate.

## Bill's Story

*Bill is a regional patient who travelled for three hours on the train to see you, and then waited for an hour and a half in clinic because you were running late. He is feeling anxious that he will miss his train home and is distracted by the unfamiliar environment of the hospital.*

*You invite Bill into your room using his name, look him in the eye, and introduce yourself with your name. When you apologise for running late, you recognise him as a human being of worth. When you invite him to take a seat and allow a few seconds for him to settle in – leaving room for him to speak, introduce his sister, and complain about the wait – you implicitly tell him that you see him, you value him and you care. You have created an opportunity to build trust. The patient doesn't owe you that trust, you have to earn it. You are using your agency and your power to create a better experience by being present, curious, and kind. You are creating the opportunity to show empathy to Bill.*

*When Bill tells you he is worried about the train, but also wants to tell you about his health, you might ask him what the best way forward is from his position, acknowledging him as integral to the consultation. If you recognise the constraints and offer to do the physical examination now and answer his most pressing questions with a follow up phone call tomorrow, you are doing more than understanding (empathy), you are actively seeking to relieve Bill's suffering (compassion). You are recognising multiple causes of suffering for Bill: his healthcare issues and his anxiety about the circumstances of his travel. You have moved from empathy to compassion.*

> **Even in times when there is no medical action that can relieve suffering, your compassion is a powerful response that is helpful for the patient and helpful for your wellbeing too.**

## FEEDBACK

Feedback is important in medicine because done well it is a great mechanism for understanding, learning, and developing your expertise. Feedback is how you know whether or not your message was understood in the way it was intended. When you were practising for your OSCEs, StAMPS, or other practical exams, you relied on feedback from others to learn how to perform well in the exam context. Feedback is also how you uncover your unconscious biases and refine your skills – clinical and non-clinical.

Feedback is a form of assessment which can make the receiver of the information feel vulnerable. Like all communication, feedback is contextual. Imagine if I said to you without warning, *"You were a bit harsh in the meeting the way you disagreed with Bridie".* If we are good friends with a high level of trust, you might laugh it off and say, *"Yeah I was, I know!",* however, if we do not know each other well, you might be affronted by my unsolicited feedback and take offence. In this state, you are likely to deny or justify, closing off any opportunity to learn from my feedback. Here again we see the importance of context to communication being effective or not.

The general purpose of feedback at work is to improve your skills so you can perform your job well. The doctors I work with have received general and broad feedback, for example:

- You're not quite ready to be a consultant yet.
- You are a bit abrupt; people don't know how to take you.
- You're not confident enough.
- Your case presentation is not succinct enough.

What do you notice about these sentences that have been given as feedback? There are three problems with these examples of feedback:

1. All of them tell the training doctor they are not enough.
2. None of them offer any suggestion about what behaviour to practise.
3. None of them are specific enough for the receiver to know how to change.

If you have received feedback like this from your supervisors, you will know that trying to interpret what you should do as a result is difficult. You are subject to your own biases and assumptions as you try to guess. Guessing is unreliable and often unhelpful – it leaves you feeling vulnerable, activating your stress response, and reducing your confidence. This kind of feedback can leave you feeling unclear about your future, confused about how significant your so-called deficit is, and what exactly you should do in order to receive a different kind of result that would demonstrate positive progress.

Tyler's Story

*Tyler received some feedback at the end of his first rotation in the ICU. His supervisor collated the feedback from various colleagues and consultants and compiled their comments into one assessment. One of the consultants said he was disorganised. Tyler did not know which consultant had said this, so couldn't ask them more about what this meant or how he could improve. There was no specific information provided about when or in what context he had been disorganised. He was not given any behavioural examples from his work and no structures or tools were offered for him to use so that he could improve. The feedback was given on his last day at the hospital, at the end of his shift and right as his supervisor was starting her shift. There was not much time to talk.*

*In the absence of specific information, this feedback is threatening to Tyler, so his brain interpreted it negatively. The whole situation was unhelpful for Tyler. He was no wiser about what was expected or how he could improve. In fact, it damaged his confidence significantly. He took most of the next rotation to regroup and work up enough courage to ask his new supervisor to help him improve how he presented at handover and manage his on-call conversations with the consultants. She told him about K-ISBAR and some other tools, which made all the difference. As a result, Tyler could take some proactive steps to improve.*

If the feedback had been behaviourally specific, Tyler would have had the opportunity to develop his practice by reflecting on his actual behaviour and measuring himself against examples given by his seniors.

An example of behaviourally specific feedback might sound something like this: *You seem disorganised at hand over. On several occasions you have told a long-winded story that seems to have no clear structure or timeline, like yesterday when you were handing over Mr Smith. It's difficult to discern what you need from me in the decision making. This has also happened when you have phoned me on call. You talk for a long time and then I still end up asking you why you are calling, which means I feel frustrated and interrupt you. What structure are you using to decide what the salient points are that I need to know?*

## GIVING FEEDBACK

Although it feels like you don't have time for this kind of conversation, remember what we have learnt about time affluence and slowing down to speed up. If you are in the privileged position of guiding young doctors, you are also in the position to influence the culture – *how we do things around here.* **The purpose of feedback at work is learning.** How you give feedback determines if learning is possible or not. If you give it with compassion and an intention to connect and support learning, you will have more impact. The system will improve over time when the collective capacity to give useful feedback lifts.

Feedback is of most value when it happens near to the event (ideally in real time), when it is behaviourally specific, and when it is given respectfully in the context of a psychologically safe place. Problems arise when feedback is given with little accountability, is vague, and is disrespectful of the person receiving the feedback. Don't store it up, share your reflections with care and respect near to the event whenever possible to maximise the learning.

Without specific behaviour-based feedback, you have no way of knowing if your message was received as you'd intended and you are blind to the unconscious messages you are sending out to others. Feedback that is designed to help people learn and is given in a supportive manner in private and with consent is powerful and can advance learning dramatically and quickly. If you have ever had a mentor 'take you under their wing', you will have experienced this kind of feedback. Care, connection, compassion, and trust enable you to develop and grow.

If you are offering feedback to a colleague, consider their psychological safety by offering a private place for the conversation whenever possible. If the feedback is difficult to share, welcome support people into the conversation and find a time that meets both of your needs. Provide feedback in a way that is strength based and empowering so that the recipient focuses on improvement rather than storing up their emotions. An impromptu doorstop conversation in the hallway is not satisfactory if the feedback is personal or challenging to hear, unless you have a very strong, trusting relationship already.

> Always ask yourself whose needs you are meeting by
> giving or withholding feedback.

Useful feedback can be given by anyone in the system. If you want to give feedback to another person, doctor or otherwise, that is designed to help them learn, develop, or improve in some way, don't expect to drop your feedback and run. Enter the conversation with the intention of holding an open, supportive dialogue and be accountable for what you say. Feedback done well is an amazing opportunity for skills-based coaching and relationship building. Follow the steps below.

1. Observe the person's behaviour and be clear in your own mind and heart what your intention is in sharing your observations.
   a. What purpose does your feedback serve?
   b. Whose needs are you serving?

2. Respectfully ask the other person's permission to share your observations with them.

3. Seek first to understand. Ask contextual questions.

4. Share your observations using specific behavioural examples, explaining what you think/feel the impact of the specific behaviour was. Stay with behavioural descriptions without judging the person or their personality.

5. Give the person time and space to process what you have said. Remember that the natural first response is to resist new information that might have previously been a blind spot. Allow the person to ask clarifying questions, think through what you have said and provide the context.

6. Discuss alternative behavioural options if the receiver is willing. If it's appropriate, share some of your own experience and be willing to revisit the conversation again.

7. Thank them for listening or sharing and encourage them to keep learning. Remember just because you have said it, doesn't mean the receiver has to use it, it's their choice.

## RECEIVING FEEDBACK

### Unsolicited

It can be difficult when unexpected feedback comes your way. Like the rest of our thinking about effective feedback, it's usually not so much about what is said, but how it's said. It can be easier to welcome feedback from someone you respect and trust because your positive regard for them buffers the experience.

If someone you do not know or do not respect offers feedback using the process outlined above, welcome it. It is not easy for people to give feedback, and they have often thought carefully about how they give it to you. Treat it as a precious gift and then actively reflect on it, perhaps talking it through with someone you trust so that you can use it to improve.

If someone offers you unsolicited and careless feedback, debrief it with someone you trust. Ruminating on it for more than a short time is not useful, why are you giving it so much credence? You need to process this kind of feedback that stays with you. What belief or bias is it triggering or unearthing? Processing out loud, either talking to someone you trust or writing about it, can often help more than endlessly thinking about it.

### Solicited

Seeking useful feedback will mean activating your personal agency and asking for it. Spend a few moments being present to yourself, be curious about what you need and why. Be kind and patient with yourself, gently recognising your own courage in working as a doctor every day. If the inner critic or imposter syndrome start making noises, acknowledge them – name them and make a values-based decision to find out what you need to know in service of your goals.

Let's try it now. Choose one area of your work you would like some feedback about.

## ACTIVITY 17

### Seeking Feedback to Learn

**Decide**: What is it you most need? What is it you want to learn about your work? What is the purpose of the feedback? What is it that you value?

**Intention**: What is your intention in asking? What do you need and what for?

**Assess**: Who is the best person to meet your need? Assess your level of safety and trust, bring someone with you if needed, work out a good time to ask – you know HALTSS will limit the person you ask – timing is important for getting the best feedback.

**Seek:** Ask them if they can help, and be specific about what you need, they can't read your mind even if it feels like they might.

**Clarify:** Ask questions to clarify meaning and to determine the behaviour that would demonstrate improvement. Ask the person giving the feedback what they recommend you do to develop in the ways they describe. Keep asking until you are clear on what to do.

**Gratitude:** Thank them for whatever insight is offered; it's not easy to give specific feedback.

## CONTINUOUS FEEDBACK BEYOND THE TRAINING YEARS

Feedback is vital if you want to improve your technical or interpersonal skills and performance. If you are no longer a trainee doctor, how do you make sure you are getting some useful and honest feedback?

> The nature of unconscious bias means you cannot accurately assess all the aspects of your work. To continuously improve your performance, you need other people whom you trust to reflect on your practice with you.

Find someone you trust and who knows your work and ask them what they have noticed about the way you communicate. Reassure them that you genuinely want to learn and grow to be a more effective communicator and acknowledge that it's hard to see yourself. Ask them to share what they have seen in terms of your actual behaviour, and to give real life examples rather than generalised statements like *you're fairly abrupt at times*. If the person giving you the feedback says something like this, ask them some follow up questions, be curious. This might sound like, *can you give me an example so I understand what I could change?*

Look for mentors, coaches, or peers with whom you can develop ongoing relationships, who can act as safe sounding boards and who can help you reflect on your practice. As you refine your communication skills, people learn to trust you more because they feel safe. High-trust relationships are the foundation of high-performance, low-conflict workplaces. In these environments, people look forward to coming to work because they feel confident that their energy will be spent on activities that they value and that means they feel productive, purposeful, and fulfilled. They have enough autonomy, agency, and meaning in their lives.

Think of effective communication as being a process of continuous improvement. Every interaction is an opportunity for you to build your skills, build trust between you and others, and increase your likelihood of influencing and effecting change, achieving your goals and expressing your agency. In this environment of effective communication, there is less energy wasted on conflict and confusion. What could you do with that available energy?

> To be truly effective and obtain maximum satisfaction and fulfilment, focus whole heartedly on *how* you communicate more than *what* you communicate. This is the essence of a 'people person' doing great work.

In your role of doctor, you have permission and influence within the healthcare system. You have a mandate to give advice and to witness vulnerability in others – you are trusted by the community. You can do great harm if you are not communicating effectively – both to your patients and to yourself. There are many risks, including misdiagnosis because you didn't hear some important information or because your patient didn't trust you enough to tell you; giving the wrong advice; being undermined by your colleagues; and not being promoted or accepted onto a training program.

These are mistakes with the potential to cause stress. You can reduce your stress and your risk by improving your communication skills. You can do this by listening better, building trust more rapidly, getting to the core of the problem more efficiently, interpreting the emotion that was limiting the outcome more accurately, being present, being curious, and being kind.

> To improve your communication, get clear on your own values and learn to regulate your emotions, otherwise your own unconscious bias and your reactive emotions will interfere with your ability to connect effectively with others.

Doctors experience high levels of burnout, suicide ideation, depression, anxiety, and stress. Healthcare is not going to change in terms of demand, distress, or disease. For doctors to be able to maintain a high level of performance, productivity, and safety for all in the short and long term, they need to be able to take good care of themselves and each other.

Compassion is a key ingredient for self and for others, especially when communication involves lots of emotion and complexity.

Understanding the emotions and values of others is a potent currency that can progress a conversation, a relationship, and health outcomes. You don't need to make wholesale changes all at once to how you communicate. You can start with any of the steps in this book.

## SUMMARY

Communication is effective when the intention is activated and understood by others. The message must be clear, concise, coherent, and understood by both sender and receiver. Agreement is not what makes it *effective*, nor is an absence of emotion indicative of effective communication. The people engaged in effective communication care about the message, the purpose, or the other people in the process. It is difficult to make communication effective when you don't care.

Effective communication creates smoother relationships because more trust is established and there is less conflict. This has a direct impact on your energy, mood, and confidence, giving you more opportunity to flourish.

Be present, curious and kind in the way you relate to others. With these three qualities, you will show you care about the others and their experience. These qualities will help you cultivate the three key skills for effective communication.

1.  Listen with your whole body.
2.  Maintain awareness.
3.  Build trust.

As you communicate in this way, you develop your skills in empathy – the ability to see the world through another person's lens. Empathy is achieved by listening deeply with the intention to understand another person's perspective, emotion and embodied experience. Empathy on its own can be a burden which activates your pain network and creates fatigue.

Compassion is the natural extension of empathic understanding. In compassion you, seek to relieve suffering. In doing so, you activate your own reward network. You can think of compassion as empathy + action. Compassionate action is a more sustainable state for you to be in neurologically as a doctor. To cultivate a compassionate stance, recognise that every time you connect with empathy and hold an intention to understand another person, this act has value and the potential to relieve the other's suffering.

Feedback is a unique gift given to another when done well. To communicate feedback effectively, treat it as an opportunity for learning, communicate effectively with care and compassion, observe specific behaviour, and offer options. Be ready to answer questions and accept that the other person will ultimately decide what they do with what you offer. Use your own agency for good. When you give and receive feedback, ask yourself, "Whose needs am I meeting?".

## Actions

- Notice who you consider to be an effective communicator. Name their skills to yourself.

- Notice who and what you care about. Does it change the way you communicate?

- Consciously set your intention on something you care about in the communication to anchor you in presence, curiosity and kindness.

- Practise listening with your whole body – tune in to your posture and open your stance.

- Be mindful.

- Recognise that building trust is an investment, smoothing communication over time.

- Notice your self-talk and cultivate compassion (not just empathy). Listening is something, sitting with someone is something, staying with the emotions in the room is something. Feel empowered to relieve suffering by connecting, one human to another.

- Give and receive feedback based on the qualities of effective communication, as if you care, as an opportunity for learning, as a gift.

# 8    CONNECT WISELY

The earlier chapters of this book have focused on your internal management, suggesting skills you can develop to look after yourself. We have progressed from the intrapersonal skills of self-regulation and stress management to the interpersonal skills of emotional intelligence and effective communication.

As you have read this book and focused on your skills of empowered agency, you have been able to reflect and connect with the ideas developed by many other people. Our lives are intricately connected, we are interdependent – from your parents and guardians taking care of you as a small child, all the way through to the people who cleaned your clinic, taught you how to palpate an abdomen, or wrote the practice guidelines for your speciality. Our drive to connect with others is embedded in our biology as a survival imperative. Without it, it is hard to flourish.

Clarity of mind and emotional intelligence are empowering skills, but for you to truly flourish, these individual skills are not enough. Seligman and other positive psychology colleagues continue to find that strong, supportive relationships are also essential for wellbeing (PERMA).

The World Health Organisation makes it very clear, "Mental health is produced socially: the presence or absence of mental health is above all a social indicator and therefore requires social, as well as individual solutions", but it's not just your mental health that is at risk if you are isolated and without close positive relationships, your physical health suffers too.

Loneliness activates your stress response. If there is no reprieve, you can be living in the red zone most of the time. Human beings are vulnerable in this state, and we know it; we become hypervigilant to threat because we feel like no one has our back.

In this chapter, I want to recognise how lonely a medical life can be and encourage you to proactively and wisely connect with others. Positive relationships are protective, enhancing your wellbeing and helping you flourish. They take care of you when you are not thriving in some way, and they facilitate good medicine, helping you reach for and achieve your potential.

> **Connecting to others wisely will help you sustain all your other efforts to be well.**

The most important function of these relationships for you as a doctor is that they facilitate a way for you to ask for help without fear of any negative professional consequences. They can be personal or professional connections; their defining feature is that they have your interests at heart.

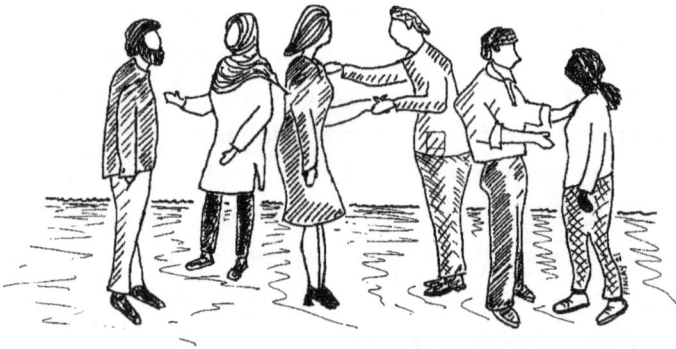

Connecting wisely is an invitation for you to be discerning about relationships and a reminder that it is wise to be well connected to those around you. Wisdom is more than understanding, wisdom is about *how* you use your knowledge and insight. Think about your existing important relationships. The kind of relationships that help you be well are meaningful, you and the other person are well aligned in your values. You don't have to agree about everything, in fact you might both value a robust debate or total blunt honesty. Every emotion is okay, or can at least be tolerated in these relationships, because the connection is bigger and more important than any one event or one experience. You value each other and the relationship you share.

If you are lucky, you will have several of these relationships. These intimate relationships generate positive emotions of hope, love, joy and gratitude. They will help to give your life it's meaning, keep you engaged, and support you to stride out into the world, believing in your own ability to achieve and contribute.

## FEELING LONELY

If you do not currently have a relationship in your life that is high in trust, start thinking about how you might deepen the connections you do have with one or two people. **What's one small act of connection you can make today?** Perhaps you can share a short conversation with your neighbour or share a little bit about what you have been watching on Netflix with someone at work.

The story you tell yourself about not having anything interesting to say or taking up people's time is nothing more than a string of words that you have chosen to believe. It may be true; it may not be true. To find out, you need to take action. Run a real-life experiment. As you do remember to practise self-compassion, go gently and kindly with the intention to learn something. You don't need a huge tribe of close connections, but you do need three or four people whom you can trust and care for, and who trust and care for you, to give yourself every opportunity to truly thrive.

Connecting with others can feel risky, especially if you haven't been practising. If you are not connected in a trusting friendship, you likely feel lonely sometimes. The truth is, many other people are lonely too. Research has found that more people are spending more time on their own than ever before, and they feel lonely. The UK government has been so concerned about the number of lonely people in their community and the requisite health problems that arise that they have appointed a Loneliness Minister.

> **Feeling lonely more than occasionally is a significant risk to your ongoing health.**

Feeling lonely is a common and normal human experience. It may or may not involve social isolation and is not the same as being alone. According to the Australian Psychological Society, one in every four people are currently experiencing loneliness. As with anything you'd like to change, you need to name it as a first step. Since it is about connection to others, your second step will be to reach out to another person. To change loneliness, you will need at least one other person's help.

After being at work with people all day, you might enjoy the opportunity to rest and recover alone in peace. However, feeling alone in your distress about work is an entirely different experience that is not okay for more than a short while. In this state, your stress response is activated, and you are less able to think clearly and creatively. Talking to someone else about your loneliness is an essential part of improving your wellbeing.

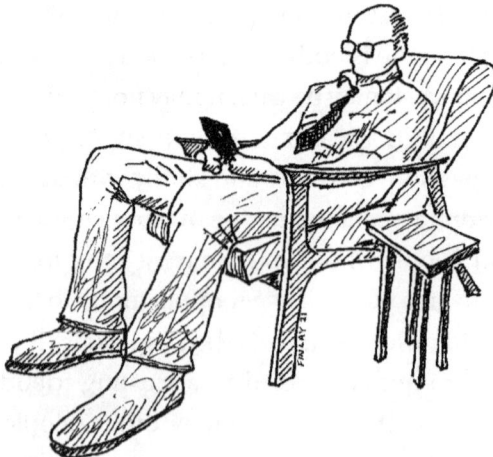

There are some simple steps you can take towards changing this:

1. Name loneliness as the problem and notice any resistance you have to sharing your experience with another person.
2. Determine what you need so that you *can* talk to someone.
3. Take action in some small way. This is vital to changing course and building supportive relationships.
4. Keep your focus on the main goal, which is to build protective relationships over time.

Starting is the most difficult part for most people. Small steps are the best way forward. Perhaps you can talk to someone on a phone helpline anonymously, or text a friend you haven't seen for a while with something simple like *how are you, it's ages since we caught up*. It doesn't have to be a deep and meaningful face-to-face conversation straight away.

You can start practising by telling someone a little bit about your experience, even if you just mention it in passing at work (*I had a pretty quiet night last night, it was a bit lonely after a week of same-same...*).

Connecting wisely is about understanding when and how to connect with others, and about who you trust. It is about using your innate need for human connection in ways that serve your ongoing wellbeing, your ability to practise great medicine, and any other goal you have. You can connect with medical colleagues and with people who have nothing to do with medicine at all, both can be protective of your wellbeing.

## Wei's Story

*Wei worked as a registrar in the ED of a big metropolitan hospital. She had a Masters of Public Health and had passed all her emergency medicine exams. She was accomplished, well regarded, and happy about her work. She was looking forward to being a consultant and thought positively about her future. She saw lots of exciting options for her career. Sadly, although her career was thriving, she was socially isolated and extremely lonely.*

*Wei lived with her brother, an engineer who was sometimes away for work. Combined with her shift work, they could go weeks without seeing each other. Their parents lived overseas. Wei talked with them several times a week. Although she had good relationships with the other members of her family, they were not accessible to her. She was very often lonely but didn't tell her parents because she didn't want them to worry. She didn't share much about her work with anyone except her immediate colleagues. Wei had never socialised with them, having only been there for nine months after doing a rural rotation the year before. Her friends from university were spread all around the country now.*

*Some of her colleagues had young children. Wei often told me in coaching how the people around her were busy, this was her way of explaining why she didn't connect with them outside her work hours. She was anxious about making new friends and told me that, "Everyone has their own lives". Wei maintained her isolation and loneliness by focusing on work, minimising her need for company and connection, and discounting her colleagues as potential options. As a result, she increased the risk of damaging her mental health and reducing her wellbeing over the longer term.*

*Many of the reasons for Wei's isolation were, if not created by her, able to be solved by her. She just needed to see this for herself. After raising her social isolation in conversation with her, I asked Wei about her previous rotation, where she had competed in triathlons. She also told me she had always wanted to try out amateur theatre after being in a play at school. These two ideas acted as a springboard for Wei. Neither of these activities were immediately possible but exposing them as ideas helped her to take some action in the service of her own wellbeing.*

*After sharing some of what we had discussed on the phone with her friend in Singapore, she found enough courage to join a local touch-football team. Conversations in coaching and with her remote friend gave her the support she needed to take care of herself better. This one step led to lots of others, including inviting one of her colleagues to join her football team. A few months later, Wei sent an email to her previous supervisor at the regional hospital where she worked the year before. He was delighted to hear from her and encouraged her to keep in touch. Wei has made a commitment to herself to do so.*

Finding the right people to connect with is not always easy and can feel like a big effort, but the return on your investment can be huge when you do. The effort you make now to find your trusted people can extend and even save your life, not just in times of strife. The effort you make often snowballs into other activities and other connections. Close relationships founded on trust and respect add richness to our lives. I encourage you to invest in some close relationships, inside and outside of medicine.

## WHO TO TRUST

Neurologically, we unconsciously decide if a new person is trustworthy rapidly and automatically – researchers estimate within three hundredths of a second. This was probably necessary on the savannah, when accurate facial recognition could save your life, but it's an overstep much of the time now. Trustworthiness is entirely contextual, changing depending on the circumstances and in relation to a person's relative feelings of power or vulnerability. Keep an open mind and use what psychologist Marsha Linehan calls your 'wise mind' to decide if you should trust a person. This state of mind integrates logical thinking and emotional awareness. In this state, you mentally step back and take some time to decide a person's trustworthiness at your own pace.

People you can trust deeply have usually proven their reliability and care. Shared high-regard builds psychological safety and respect. Look at the people you already trust, what is it that you value about them? What qualities have they demonstrated that have shown you they are trustworthy? Use these reflections to guide your decisions. There is some risk in deciding to trust another person. The risk in not trusting anyone is worse when it comes to taking good care of yourself.

## RELATIONSHIPS ARE PROTECTIVE

Harvard has been conducting a longitudinal study for 83 years asking what makes people happy. They have concluded that the most important factor for people to be happy and healthy is *good relationships*. Three key findings support their conclusion:

1. **Loneliness shortens lifespan.** Participants who were isolated and lonely were less happy. Their health and their brain function declined earlier than those who were not lonely.
2. **Warm, loving relationships are protective.** Relationships that are affectionless and contentious have negative impacts on health and happiness.
3. **Good relationships are good for the brain.** Participants who were in a relationship where they knew someone supported them had sharper memories for longer.

Further research published in '*Perspectives on Psychological Science*' concluded that prolonged isolation has the equivalent negative health effects as smoking 15 cigarettes a day. An earlier study found that subjective feelings of loneliness increased the risk of mortality between 26 - 45%. John Cacioppo and his colleagues have dedicated their careers to researching and understanding loneliness, which Johann Hari outlines in his book '*Lost Connections*.' Cacioppo concludes that "Evolution has shaped us to feel bad in isolation and to feel insecure" as a means of forcing us back to the group. You will remember that one of the key PERMA factors for wellbeing is positive relationships. We need each other.

## CONNECTING TO COLLEAGUES AT WORK

Gallup has consistently found that having a best friend at work significantly improves people's performance. For example, women who strongly agree they have a best friend at work are more than twice as likely to be engaged (63%) compared with the women who say otherwise (29%). This is of significance, considering 70% of the global healthcare workforce are women. In 2017, almost half of doctors in OECD countries were women. In Australia in 2016, 41% of doctors were women.

More generally, Gallup has found that employees stay at organisations with exceptional workplace cultures. Cultures characterised by overall feelings of trust, belonging and inclusion. In other words, work-places that meet our basic psychological needs for safety, belonging, and autonomy instil loyalty in their staff. People enjoy interacting with each other. Competitiveness and perfectionism do not foster this kind of culture.

Gallup concludes that people want to create meaningful connec-tions and that organisations who create cultures where friendships can naturally develop and thrive will see the benefits in terms of engagement and performance.

## YOUR RELATIONSHIPS

Can you call to mind the relationships you have, or have had, where you feel warmly welcomed and your psychological needs for safety, belong-ing, and autonomy are met? It's easy to give your energy to these relation-ships; they enhance your life because they are high in trust. Inside these relationships, you are free to learn, test your ideas, and make mistakes.

Now think about your relationships within medicine. Do you have a mentor, trusted advisor, or confidant anywhere within your profession? I usually ask new coaching clients this question. The vast majority of doc-tors I work with tell me they have a mentor or someone who has encour-aged them in their medical journey. Then I ask them if they are currently in contact with this person, how they catch up and how often. The major-ity are not in contact and are not sure if they could reach out to the person they think of as their mentor.

### Reflection

- Is this you too?
- What caused your disconnection from this person whom you regard so highly?
- If another doctor considered you to be a positive mentor or some sort of trusted guide, would you welcome their keeping in touch, even if you no longer worked together?

Your answers to these three questions may give you some direction. Perhaps you would like to reconnect with someone you've previously worked with, either as their mentor or because you think of them as a mentor. Maybe your answers to these three questions give you some insight into another facet of medical culture. Is it okay to keep in touch with your mentors, or are they only ever allowed to be temporary relationships? If you would not be comfortable reaching out to someone you had a good working relationship with in the past, can you dig a little deeper and ask yourself why not?

## ACTIVITY 18

Most of the doctors I talk to about their mentors say they don't keep in touch because the mentor is busy, and they don't want to take up their time. If this is your answer too, I have eight more questions for you to consider:

1. Do you value human connection with other doctors?
2. What specifically do you value about this human connection?
3. How does your answer to the previous question add to your life and your practice of medicine?
4. How does the story of "they are busy or important" serve you?
5. What does this story have you saying about yourself?
6. Do you really believe that story about yourself?
7. What does the story about yourself have you doing?
8. Does that serve your goals for medicine, your patients or your own life?

## BELONGING TO MEDICINE

Medicine has a strong culture of belonging. Doctors identify staunchly with their profession and feel a bond born out of the shared difficult circumstances they graduate through in the early years of their training. Doctors across the world share a genuine respect for each other's commitment.

> However, belonging is dependent on maintaining the social norms, especially the code of silence if you are not coping.

A profound contradiction exists: although doctors belong to the same 'club', they often cannot be honest with each other about how they are or are not coping. This is because of the ongoing competition between them and the fear and stigma of being judged as weak or not up to the job. This requirement to maintain the status quo, a veneer of coping at all costs, and to keep competing can make medicine an extremely isolating profession.

In addition, you have probably moved constantly throughout your training years in pursuit of speciality training and opportunity. Separated from family and friends, working long hours, and studying for much longer than your peers in other professions, you have probably had very little time for a social life. Harvard Business Review published a survey in 2018 that found doctors to be one of the loneliest of professional workers.

> Strong supportive relationships will help you to sustain your individual efforts.

Knowing you have people who will encourage you and not judge you facilitates experimentation, allowing you to challenge yourself and giving you a forum to share your concerns.

Sustaining a medical career on your own is impossible. Nearly every part of your work relies on someone else to make it happen. Surgeons need anaesthetists and technicians, physicians need nursing support, medical researchers do their work in a long chain of experiments undertaken by other people. In truth, the idea that you ever *do* medicine alone is ignoring all those who have helped you get this far, including the patients.

## FIND YOUR TRIBE

Chapter 4 of this book pointed you to the importance of meaning and purpose in your life. Sharing that purpose with others who care about it like you do amplifies your ability to advance your cause. We understand our causes by telling each other stories. It's the story you tell that another person emotionally connects to. They believe in the story.

Seth Godin describes a tribe as a group of people with a shared interest and a way to communicate. A tribe can vary in size. In leadership literature, it usually refers to 20 to 150 people. The members of a tribe have a shared purpose. The key emotion for any tribe is care – caring for each other as a community and caring for the shared purpose. Do you have a community of people you belong to where you share a purpose that you care deeply about, and where you care about the other members of the community?

This is not about networking; it's about being very clear on what you care about and connecting to that in committed ways. It is about being cared about by others who share your values and purpose, and it is about having confidence that someone has your back. You do not need to be a perfect, endlessly resilient, competing robot. The patients don't want you to be, they know and trust that you are competent. They want to know you care. Your loved ones don't need you to be 110% committed to medicine, they are already proud of you. They want to connect with you whole heartedly.

In order to choose your tribes wisely, you will need to take some risks and possibly do some things you haven't felt willing to do before. It will take some effort. The stable internal environment you have been learning to cultivate in the earlier chapters will guide you. Hold your meaning, intention, and values in the front of your mind, feel whatever emotions arise and respond skilfully. I know you can do it; I've had the privilege of witnessing many other doctors walk along this path.

When you find your tribe, you will be able to be vulnerable; freely express your needs and desires; and ask for what you need, knowing that you will not be judged and help will be readily available. In these tribes, you are deeply valued. Your positive emotions increase, improving your immune function, reducing your stress, and enabling you to live a truly meaningful life.

Our program *Recalibrate* is creating a tribe of doctors who believe in taking better care of themselves and each other. They come together around a common belief that they can learn the skills to take better care of themselves and that doing so will result in providing better healthcare for their patients. Their purpose is clear, and they have the means to communicate together in service of that purpose. The *Recalibrate* community is one tribe, but there are many, and you can initiate your own too. A tribe works with shared values and shoots for a noble cause. ***Recalibrate's*** **noble cause is a healthcare system that prioritises doctor wellbeing first**, knowing that patients will inevitably benefit.

Do you feel part of a medical tribe either in your speciality or in your organisation? What is the benefit for you of belonging to your tribe?

## ASKING FOR HELP

Psychologists from Columbia University conducted a study in which people asked strangers in New York City if they could use their phone to make a call – that's it, no justification or explanation. Many strangers said yes. On average, it took only two requests. Before each variation of this study (including one where participants asked strangers for money), the researchers asked the participants to estimate how many people they would need to approach before they were successful. In every variation, participants underestimated others' willingness and ability to help.

> People want to help you much more often than you think they do.

Doctors are reluctant to ask for help. This is normal in a competitive environment like medicine. Do you worry that there will be a social cost of seeking help? This belief is common in healthcare. It goes something like this: *If I ask for help, I am admitting that I am weak, ignorant, incapable, lazy or dependant, so I won't ask.*

Is this what you do? Are you worried about your reputation or about being rejected? These are painful experiences when they do happen, your brain is trying to protect you. In doing so you limit your opportunity to learn, even to impress. This social norm is a powerful force and continues to exist in people's minds as a belief even though it might be irrational at times. People are willing and able to help if you let them. When was the last time you asked anyone for help in your life?

Under the right circumstances, asking for help can positively add to others' perception of your capacity. Asking for help can demonstrate:

- your confidence
- your respect for the other person's capability and knowledge
- your wisdom in discerning your need for help
- that you are willing to take risks.

You need to be discerning though, if you ask a simple lazy question, you will be judged swiftly as exactly that. How do you know when to ask? Use the skills you have been reading about here.

- ✓ Be mindful
- ✓ Make values-based decisions
- ✓ Develop your emotional intelligence
- ✓ Be thoughtful about how you communicate
- ✓ Build strong, trusting relationships.

Perception is important when you are asking for help. Ask people you trust, people who are perceptive about your wisdom in knowing when to ask, and those who can actually help you. Having one rule that says never to ask for help is cognitively rigid and unhelpful. If you never ask for help, does that mean you know everything there is to know and can do every-thing already? Asking questions or asking for help can demonstrate trust and inspire others. It may not be the sin medicine has made it out to be.

People who don't ask for help are basing their decision on fear. Few successful doctors advanced their medical career without help from someone, you just may not have seen it. Asking for a senior's help can be a sign of respect. The mindset of inconveniencing them is not helpful. Be thoughtful about your questions and the timing, and reframe asking for help to be more internally useful. For example, focus on a story such as: you are asking to ensure the patient gets the best possible care, or to ensure that you are growing in your skills and capacity. When the other person helps you, express your gratitude and keep moving. Rumination serves no one.

Build relationships with your colleagues constantly, you never know who can help you. People are more likely to help you if they regard you positively – make friends and have friendly relations as much as possible, remembering the practice of *just like me* is helpful in generating a positive attitude towards others. Consider the possible outcomes if you don't ask, don't wait until it's too late. Be proactive. Start by asking people you are comfortable and confident with, it's fine if that means asking your friends and family, you are practising.

## PLEASE DON'T SUFFER ALONE

The worst outcome of a person not asking for help and not trusting anyone with their story is suicide. Besides the fun and personal enrichment of diverse connections, this is the main reason to have a medical tribe and a non-medical tribe. If you are not able to share your experience at work because of shame, fear about reputation, or maintaining the code of silence, then tell someone outside of medicine – a coach, your GP, your best friend, sibling or parent, a counsellor, or a helpline counsellor. Remember that your relationship with someone who loves you or cares about you is bigger than any feeling or story you hold.

Doctors often keep their emotional burden secret from their families because they don't want their loved ones to worry. Many doctors I know are conscious not to bring too much doom and gloom home from work. You also need to maintain your patients' confidentiality. Keeping a boundary around the content of your work is an attempt to protect yourself and an effort to keep work from seeping into the sanctuary of your home.

The problem is, if you can't trust anyone at work with your emotions and your worries for fear of being tarnished, and you can't tell your loved ones out of a desire to protect them from distress, who can you share your stories with? Giving voice to your stories is vital for your wellbeing and mental health.

> The last invitation in this book is to invite you to be truly accountable for your wellbeing by committing to practising asking for help.

Nominate your safe trusted people so that you can start sharing some of your stories with them. If you don't have those people yet, your commitment is to find them and start fostering these relationships. Enlist the help of a coach, psychologist, or the chaplain at work. Honour your GP in their role as your primary care person and let them care for you, it is their specialty. You are responsible for building a consistent and long term partnership with them; they want to support you and help you to be well.

## REGRETS

Bronnie Ware is an Australian nurse and author who worked in palliative care. In her book '*Regrets of the Dying*', she recognises the five common regrets people tend to express in the last stages of their life. The regrets touch upon being more genuine, not working so hard, expressing true feelings, staying in touch with friends, and finding more joy in life.

The developmental work I have encouraged in this book is partly designed to help you take the action you need to minimise the risk of having these regrets in your life. While 'staying in touch with friends' may be the most obvious in relation to this chapter, all of these regrets may be ameliorated if you connect openly with others and truly engage in building high-trust relationships. Of course, you will not trust everyone. To be well you need to feel connected to a few positive supportive people in your life who will look out for you because they want to, because they care.

You need to be able to recognise when you need to ask for their help. Just as you don't need to be with your close friends all the time, you don't need to be asking for help all the time, but as you practise, you may find you want to. The more you cultivate deep trusting friendships and the more you collaborate and ask for help, the more comfortable you will be. As you practise your skills, you will become more discerning and wiser about how you connect with those around you.

Prioritise your connections with your loved ones, make more time for them. Find at least two or three other people you can trust and share your concerns with, inside and outside medicine. Intentionally and consciously cultivate these relationships. Don't wait. You are not an island, if you are behaving like one you are risking your current and future wellbeing.

## DESIGN YOUR OWN BEST LIFE

In coaching, we ask a lot of powerful questions. Two important ones are:

1. Who do you want to be?
2. What do you want your life to be about?

How do you answer these questions? Take a moment to answer them.

Did you say anything that *relates* to others? Maybe you want to be a role model to younger doctors or to your children. Perhaps you want to take the stigma out of mental illness. Perhaps you want to always keep some fun in your life. There are very few things you can be and do that don't relate to other people.

What's the worst thing that can happen if you get up close and personal with one or two other people?

What do you need from the people around you, as a human being and as a doctor, so that you can thrive?

There are many things to challenge your wellbeing and focus on when you work in medicine. Over time, work to find your tribe, that group of people with whom you share a common purpose and with whom you want to communicate about that purpose. Tribes are exciting, they make new things happen. Better still, find a couple of tribes that you can actively participate in and feel an abundance of belonging and safety. It's up to you, and it's totally worth it.

## SUMMARY

1.  Your wellbeing and survival are dependent on good relationships with others.
2.  Build a few close relationships, they are protective of your mental health.
3.  Foster friendships inside and outside of medicine.
4.  Find the tribe of people who care about what you care about and they will also care about you.
5.  People generally want to help others.
6.  Practise asking for help in good times so it's easier to do in hard times.
7.  People perceive others who ask for help as wise and trustworthy.
8.  Commit to practising your interpersonal skills and to asking for help.
9.  Foster an open, trusting partnership with a GP who you see regularly.

* * *

If you are in distress and do not know who to call, phone Lifeline or Docs4Docs. Over 1 million people in Australia do every year. You may not know it, but there are *always* places for listening and people there whose expertise is in caring, careful listening. You can remain anonymous and start getting the help you need. Use the resources listed at the end of the book (p. 295) and visit www.coachingfordoctors.net.au for an updated list. Most Colleges and medical agencies around the world can help you find the support you need. If you are unsure start by talking with your primary care physician.

# 9 SUSTAIN BALANCE

*"Life is a choice. It is YOUR life.*
*Choose consciously, choose wisely, choose honestly.*
*Choose happiness."*
*— Bronnie Ware*

Your fulfilling life is defined by you. Broadly speaking, it is one that has meaning, purpose and value to you. Doctors often say they want a more balanced life. Depending on where you are in your career, different activities will bring you balance. Wherever you are in your medical journey, you need to attend to both ends of your seesaw if you want to achieve balance. A thriving life includes everything life offers, it's not about having everything that is good, positive and easy. It's about having the skills and resources you need to respond effectively with confidence, patience and love. It's about feeling empowered enough within your own life to maintain your balance enough of the time. How much is enough for you will determine your level of satisfaction. **Go for excellence rather than perfection**, and find a great coach to help you.

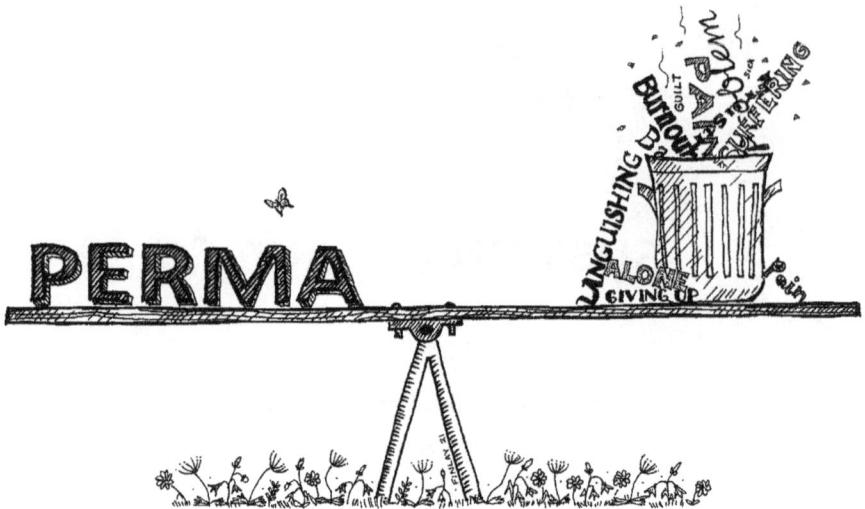

To thrive, you will need to proactively attend to the end of the seesaw where the problems and the pain sit. No matter how well you can describe your pain/problem, only knowing about that end will keep you tumbling to the ground. To change your experience, you need to give some attention and energy to the PERMA end. Here's a quick reminder of what's on the other end to help you flourish:

1.  **Positive emotion** – feeling happiness, pleasure, comfort, and a sense of life satisfaction
2.  **Engagement** – being in a state of flow as assessed subjectively by the experiencer
3.  **Relationships** – feeling connected: we are social animals and do better in each other's company
4.  **Meaning** – belonging to and serving something bigger than yourself
5.  **Accomplishment** – having a sense of achievement and progress in your chosen activity.

> You must understand the stressors in your life as well as what brings you meaning and joy. Maintaining awareness and paying attention to both is everyday forever work.

There is a considerable research base about how adults grow and develop. With each stage of development, an adult's relationship to their life, to others, and to their work changes. Each stage incorporates the previous step and adds new capacity. What you focus on – the problem, the outcome, the process, your own state – will affect if you feel and believe yourself to be empowered or powerless. The way you author your own story is different at each stage of development. As you attend to what truly matters in your life and confront the belief structures and biases that undermine you, your capacity grows.

Belief systems are the software of our brain driving the conclusions we make about ourselves, others, and our organisations. Mindfulness skills give us the capacity to notice what is happening. Clarity of mind, emotional intelligence, compassion, a trusted community, and a willingness to ask for help are the skills we use to design a better way.

Welcome your whole life with compassion. Every experience – thoughts, emotions, sensations. These are your teachers. Sit with them, listen deeply for their wisdom. Stop rushing around, numbing and ignoring yourself to what is already here. The wisdom you need is in your body. To hear it, you will need to be still and open your heart and mind. To be well, you need to value it enough to make a little bit of effort every day. Enough to inquire:

- Who am I?
- What do I want?
- What do I need?

When you experience something that triggers a core belief, uncovers a blind spot, or has you feeling vulnerable, consider it a gift. Use the space between the stimulus and your response to choose. Feel your own agency and recognise it as an opportunity to learn and discover. Beliefs are reinforcing, we select the data that maintains them without even trying. Expose your autopilot, welcome it – gosh it makes you efficient. Then decide if it's efficiency or effectiveness you're going for in each particular situation.

Sustaining this kind of gentle enquiry, maintaining your curiosity in the face of so many patients, so much organisational pressure, so much cultural expectation, and so much perfectionism is difficult. It's helpful to have others around you who share this purpose. Build your own community of trust and practise asking for help in small and large tasks and in understanding yourself. Don't wait until your back is against the wall – we care about you. We want to help; we want to feel connected. Positive relationships are key to wellbeing and longevity. Remember you are human; your self is more important than any role, including that of doctor. Human beings thrive on compassionate connection.

Practising the intra- and interpersonal skills described in this book will go a long way in helping you build positive relationships, in being well, and in having a sustainable medical career that is fulfilling. As you find or grow your own sense of self, your voice and your power, directing your energy in ways that you care about, you are more likely to make an impact on the system. Your chances are much greater if you have done the work on yourself first. Look inward. Practice using your energy well, respond skilfully internally and eternally.

> Remember to breathe out long and slow, often.
> Make your self-talk full of compassion to activate your reward circuits.
> Call empathy fatigue by its right name.
> Slow down to speed up.

We have covered a lot of ground in *The Thriving Doctor*.

Where will you place your focus as you start to take better care of yourself?

Choose one or two practices from the summary on the final page. Start small but commit to practising every day. Build an accountability process by telling someone else what you are practising. Keep a note in your journal and engage a coach, psychologist, counsellor, or member of your peer group. Most of all, keep practising with kindness towards yourself. The work you do is complex, challenging and often risky, give yourself the best chance of success by collaborating openly with others. You can thrive in medicine and the people around you will also benefit. **Lean in, *you're worth it.***

## 32 SKILLS DOCTORS CAN PRACTISE TO HELP THEM THRIVE

1. Prioritise sleeping for 7 to 9 hours in every 24.
2. Develop a daily mindful practice, breathe.
3. Grow your emotional literacy by noticing your bodily sensations and naming your emotions. Learn to welcome all emotions.
4. Remember you have unconscious bias, grow your self-awareness. Ask others to help you and practise *Just Like Me.*
5. Use compartmentalising as a short-term strategy only, tell someone you trust about the difficulties in your work and the impact they have on you.
6. Clarify your meaning and purpose and use these to anchor your decisions.
7. Clarify your beliefs and values to help you grow into your best self.
8. Understand that you are not your role. Who are you? What do you want?
9. Recognise and name your stressors.
10. Welcome your body's efficient *activation* as it responds to threat (red zone).
11. Actively prioritise activities that help your body to engage the relaxation response (green zone).
12. Say to yourself: I'm practising getting comfortable with being uncomfortable (stop numbing, suppressing, and ignoring your experiences).
13. Practise acceptance instead of rumination.
14. Defuse from your thoughts – you are not your thoughts.
15. Reframe time, think about energy instead.

16. Give your energy to that which you can control, your circle of influence.
17. Learn the skills of self-compassion and practise often.
18. Practise gratitude every day to bring balance to your mind and life.
19. Attend to your emotional habits, are they serving you well?
20. Notice when you approach and avoid your emotions and your life. Activate your conscious choice.
21. Address anxiety, guilt, shame, and any other sticky emotion by seeking help. Learn how to manage them.
22. Plan your first action for 'hot' moments so you can respond to them instead of falling back on autopilot reactions that are inflammatory.
23. Decide to improve your communication skills. Start by committing to *seek first to understand.*
24. Listen with care, connection, presence, curiosity, kindness, empathy and trust.
25. Listen with your whole body.
26. Practise compassion as much as possible, it's good for others and for you.
27. Give and receive feedback with an intention to create learning.
28. Value and cultivate strong healthy relationships on purpose.
29. Create or join a tribe that shares a purpose you hold dear to your heart.
30. Ask for help often, it builds connection, trust and respect.
31. Cultivate a strong partnership with a GP who you can have an ongoing trusting relationship with.
32. Prioritise your loved ones, make more time to be with them and be present.

May you be well!
XS

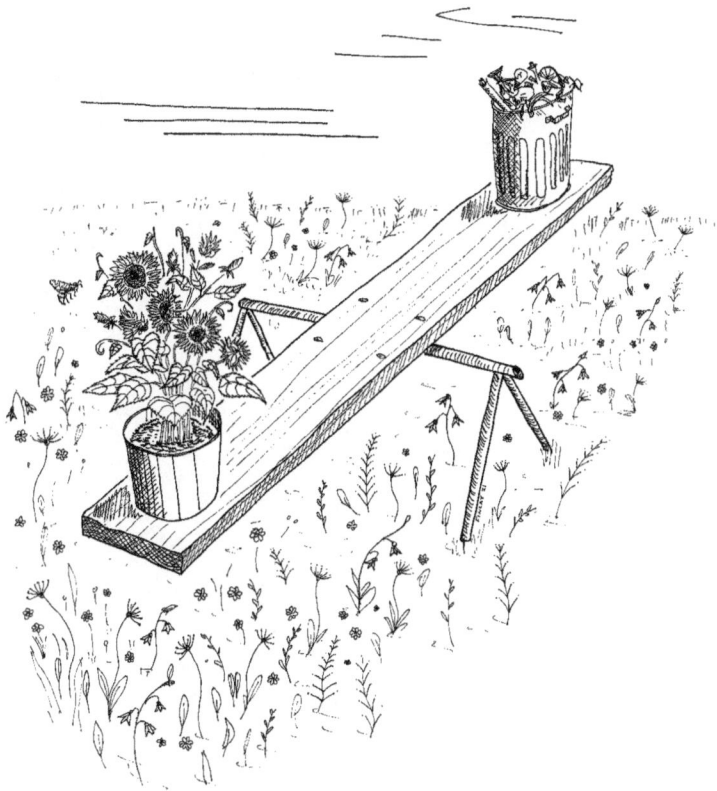

# EPILOGUE

Doctors constantly ask me why I care about doctor wellbeing. It's deeply personal. I do have doctors in my family who I love, but that's not why I do this work. In 2007, the realities of healthcare came home to me in a raft of new ways, when my husband Tim was diagnosed with cholangiocarcinoma. He was thirty-eight, while our children were only three, five and six years old.

For four years, I learnt about the healthcare system from the other side, as a person walking closely with someone who has cancer, a patient. The perspective was so different from the one I held working as a psychologist. During those four years Tim was well much of the time, returning to full time work and even successfully achieving a new CEO role. He was also literally on death's doorstep, spending eleven days in ICU in an induced coma after his first chemotherapy. Life was absolutely a rollercoaster. Tim's diagnosis was diabolical for our family, changing everything, and in 2011 he died. That's still hard to say.

Tim had many, many stays in various hospitals. There were new treatments, adjunct therapies, and hundreds of different healthcare workers. We experienced the full spectrum of emotions, learning to manage the extremes of grief, threat, anger, relief, sadness, exhilaration, and distress. Three things anchored us - mindfulness, crystal clear values, and accepting help. These anchors meant we could meet any emotion, maintain some energy and some stability, and engage our own autonomy. We felt deeply connected to those who mattered.

As a psychologist, I might have had a head start, but nothing prepared me for this journey. I had to learn the skills I needed to take care of myself, so that I could take care of Tim and our children.

During those four years, many of the emotions I experienced were triggered by the healthcare system, more specifically by individual providers – doctors and nurses from several specialties, allied health practitioners including counsellors, chaplains, physiotherapists, a nutritionist, dietician, herbalist, massage therapists, chiropractors, other hospital staff like cleaners, caterers, security, administrators.

In these people we met the full continuum of human wellness. Some healthcare workers were obviously grounded and energised, warm and kind, actively interested in what we needed and how we were, eager to explain to us the why, how or what of what was happening. Others were at the opposite end of the continuum, oblivious to the impact of their terse words, their unavailability, or their impatience on us. Sometimes we witnessed this disengaged, even hostile 'care' of other patients and sadly we were also exposed to conflict and disrespect between healthcare worker colleagues.

I was so angry during those years about some of the doctors and nurses we met. Most allied health and adjunct therapists seemed to be present and focused on Tim and his needs, but many of the doctors and nurses were not. They seemed to always be in a hurry, more often looking at their watches and the door than Tim, frustrated by our questions. There was rarely a sense of partnership when Tim was in hospital, more a sense of being done to, ticked off the list, handballed to the next person.

It was a relief to visit Tim's GP or his herbalist, who always gave us time, listened carefully and asked thoughtful questions. Both the GP and the herbalist had built a relationship with Tim and with me. We trusted them, these conversations did not induce anxiety. Even though the subject matter was heavy, we felt safe, seen and cared for. Our energy was available for thinking, healing, connecting and making progress.

I understood the doctors and nurses had done everything medical science could to extend Tim's life and take care of him. On that front they did an extraordinary job and we remain forever grateful to them. I now know that most of these doctors and nurses were doing the best they could. In truth, their gruffness was probably rarely about us.

Still, meeting some of the doctors had taken an emotional toll on Tim and I. Doctors were almost always the decision makers, they held the knowledge we sought and the structural power. There were too many times that we felt under threat, our stress response amplified by our interactions with, or lack of access to doctors. Our energy was often used on managing these relationships instead of on our own precious wellbeing.

After Tim died, I reflected on what I had learnt about healthcare from this new perspective of patient family. As a psychologist, executive coach and meditation teacher, I wondered what I could do to help patients have a better experience. Coming into the healthcare system as a family learning about cancer had been so disorienting. Everything had seemed outside of our control, everything felt threatening not only to Tim's life, but to the safety of our whole family, to our collective future. Like so many people after a personal tragedy, I wanted to do something useful with what I had experienced, to make the loss of Tim mean something.

I knew I had a lot to learn. I started talking to doctors, including some of those who had looked after Tim. I wanted to understand what life was like as a doctor. Was it like other jobs that just became routine and boring after a while? How did doctors cope with all this bad news and distress they immersed themselves in day after day? Why did they do the things they did? I wanted to understand what was included in medical training. Did doctors learn about communication, compassion, human motivation and emotional intelligence. Were my expectations unrealistic?

The more questions I asked and conversations I had, the more curious I became. Until eventually, I learnt so much about being a doctor that I morphed into an advocate for doctors! That is not what I expected to happen. I had started from a place of 'othering' doctors, but the more I learnt the more I found out that we are the same. It has been a powerful lesson in my own life of 'seek first to understand'. Life is full of surprises. My curiosity and desire for better patient care has led me to coaching doctors, learning from them, and seeking ways to build a healthcare system that is better for everyone, beginning with doctors.

Over the course of the past ten years, I have had the great fortune to be involved in several healthcare movements, beginning with my own attempt at bringing people together at the Gippsland Health Summits in 2015 and 2017. This was truly heartfelt work that I poured my heart and soul into in the early years without Tim, and many blessings have since poured from there.

Of particular note, it was through this vision that I met Professor Catherine Crock, Dr Vijay Roach, Professor Munjed Al Muderis and Dr Helena Popovic. The impact of these busy leading doctors being willing to travel to a rural town to join me in my cause – to bring healthcare providers and the public together to learn about how to improve healthcare – simply because I asked them to, cannot be adequately measured. These four extraordinary people gave me the confidence that I could contribute something worthwhile, that I could have a voice and make a difference to patient care, and as it turns out, to doctor care.

Since then, I have had the joy and fortune to be part of planning and delivering six years of Gathering of Kindness events, attended two Compassion Revolution conferences and this year presented at the first Ending Physician Burnout Global Summit. Healthcare is transforming. We are relearning the value of human connection as a treatment in and of itself. We recognise care, compassion and human connection as a survival imperative, and I am now truly optimistic about the future of healthcare.

This is not a book about burnout, and I hope that was clear as you read it. The Thriving Doctor is about prevention and early intervention. When doctors are well and well cared for, all other healthcare goals are more attainable. We all benefit.

Test readers of *The Thriving Doctor* asked me to comment on gallows humour as a coping strategy, how to 'manage up', how to respond effectively to difficult HR processes and inadequate or poor management, how to stop bullying and discriminatory practices and many more specific topics. All issues I work with every day with doctors in coaching. The skills I have invited you to build will help you respond to these complex issues more effectively.  Do the work of personal development, responsibility and accountability, build your support network. I hope you will join us as we collectively activate our agency, working to build a much better healthcare system.

The work I do with doctors is about living a life on purpose. Set your intention, live with meaning, make the effort to learn the skills you need to enjoy your life, get the right people around you to help you make a consistent effort to be well. You're worth it, but you have to believe it yourself. Make the effort, be the best doctor you can be, for *your* sake as much as anyone else's.

Thank you to every doctor and to every person who works in healthcare. It is my honour and privilege to walk with you.

# REFERENCES

## Introduction

1.  Pearl, R.*Uncaring: How the culture of medicine kills doctors and patients.* New York: Public Affairs (Hfatchett Book Group), 2021

2.  Dewar, B, Charmel, P.A., Guastello, S. and Frampton, S.B. "Compassion in Action." *The Putting Patients First Field Guide* (2013): 69-89

3.  Haslam, N. "Humanising Medical Practice: The Role of Empathy." *Medical Journal of Australia* (2007): 187(7), 381-82

4.  Hojat, M., Louis, D.Z., Markham, F.W., Wender, R and others. "Physicians' Empathy and Clinical Outcomes for Diabetic Patients." *Academic Medicine* (2011): 86(3), 359-364

5.  Malloy, R. and J. Otto. "A Steady Dose of Empathy." *Hospital and Health Networks Daily* (June 7 , 2012)

6.  Mulley Jnr, A.G. and J.E. Wennberg (2011) *Reducing Unwarranted Variation in Clinical Practice by Supporting Clinicians and Patients in Decision Making. In Better Doctors, Better Patients, Better Decisions. Ed.Gigerenzer, G and Muir Gray, J.A.* Massachusetts: The MIT Press, 2011.

7.  "Norcross and Lambert compendium of evidence-based relationships." *Psychotherapy in Australia* Vol 19, No. 3 (May 2013)

8.  Ovretveit, J. *Do Changes to Patient-Provider Relationships Improve Quality and Save Money? Vol 1: Summary of a Review of the Evidence.* London: Health Foundation, 2012

9.  Rakel, D.P., et. al. "Perception of Empathy in the Therapeutic Encounter: Effects on the Common Cold." *Patient Education and Counselling* (2011): 85(3), 390-397

10. Rakel, D.P., et. al. "Practitioner Empathy and the Duration of the Common Cold." *Family Medicine* (2009): 41(7), 494-501

11. Stewart, MA. "Effective physician-patient communication and health outcomes: A review." *CMAJ* (1995): 152(9), 1423-33.

12. Beach MC, Keruly J, Moore RD. "Is the quality of the patient-provider relationship associated with better adherence and health outcomes for patients with HIV?" *J Gen Intern Med* (2006): 21(6):661-5.

13. DiMatteo, MR. "Enhancing patient adherence to medical recommendations." *JAMA* (1994): 271(1):79-83.

14. DiMatteo MR, Sherbourne CD, Hays RD, et al. "Physicians' characteristics influence patients' adherence to medical treatment: Results from the Medical Outcomes Study." *Health Psychol* (1993): 12(2):93-102.

15. Institute of Medicine, Crossing the Quality Chasm, 2001 National Academy Press

16. Shanafelt, Tait D., et. al. "American Medical Association, Creating a Resilient Organisation." https://www.ihf-fih.org/wordpress/wp-content/uploads/2021/02/caring-for-health-care-workers-covid-19.pdf. Accessed May, 2020.

17. Christine Sinsky MD Vice President, Professional Satisfaction AMA and Internist in Private Practice discusses the impact of leadership and 20% of doing what gives you joy at work for the Research Medical Library at University of Texas MD Anderson Cancer Center 25-27 September 2017. https://www.youtube.com/watch?v=POZvCRdNbI8

18. Christine Sinsky MD, FACP Vice President, Professional Satisfaction AMA and Internist in Private Practice. 25x5 Presentation Plenary Talk for Convergent Actions, 23 Feb 2021. https://www.youtube.com/watch?v=_6K2wSggZVM

## Chapter 1

19. https://gordonlegal.com.au/services/class-actions/victorian-doctors-class-action/
https://amavic.com.au/news---resources/victorian-doctors-class-action

20. McEwan, K. *Resilience at Work, A Framework for Coaching and Interventions.*

21. https://workingwithresilience.com.au/wp-content/uploads/2018/09/Whitepaper-Sept18.pdf

22. Emotions are present in everything:

    Kahneman, D. *Thinking, Fast and Slow.* New York: Farrar, Straus and Giroux, 2011.

    Davidson R. and Begley, S. *The Emotional Life of the Brain.* London: Hodder and Stoughton, 2013.

23. Hard wired to connect: some excellent resources for you to use on this topic

    https://dana.org/article/in-sync-how-humans-are-hard-wired-for-social-relationships/

    https://findingmastery.net/andrew-huberman/

    https://drsarahmckay.com/theneuroscienceacademy/

24. The hidden curriculum in undergraduate medical education: qualitative study of medical students' perceptions of teaching BMJ 2004;329:770. https://www.bmj.com/content/329/7469/770

    The Contemporary Hidden Curriculum in Medical Education. Vijay Rajput, Anuradha Lele Mookerjee, Consuelo Cagande 9/12/2017. https://www.mededpublish.org/manuscripts/1193

Cowell, Richard N. The hidden curriculum: a theoretical framework and a pilot study. Cambridge: Harvard Graduate School of Education, 1972

25. Riess, Helen, MD, et. al. "Empathy Training for Resident Physicians: A Randomized Controlled Trial of a Neuroscience-Informed Curriculum." *J Gen Intern Med (2012): 27(10): 1280-126.* https://www.ncbi.nlm.nih.gov/pmc/articles/PMC3445669/

26. Hojat, Mohammadreza, PhD, et. al. "Does Empathy Decline in the Clinical Phase of Medical Education? A Nationwide, Multi-Institutional, Cross-Sectional Study of Students at DO-Granting Medical Schools. *Academic Medicine* Vol. 95, Issue 6. (2020): 911-918. https://journals.lww.com/academicmedicine/fulltext/2020/06000/does_empathy_decline_in_the_clinical_phase_of.39.aspx

27. Thomas, Matthew R., et. al. "How do distress and well-being relate to medical student empathy? A multicenter study." *General Internal Medicine* (2007): 22(2):177-83. https://pubmed.ncbi.nlm.nih.gov/17356983/

28. Gerada, C. "Doctors, suicide and mental illness." *BJPsych Bull.* (2018): 42(4): 165–168. https://www.ncbi.nlm.nih.gov/pmc/articles/PMC6436060/

29. Occupational Health and Safety Risk in Public Hospitals, Victorian Auditor General Report 2013. https://www.parliament.vic.gov.au/file_uploads/21031128-OHS-in-Hospitals_WvtQ97LM.pdf

30. Bullying and Harassment in the Health Sector, Victorian Auditor General Report 2016. https://www.audit.vic.gov.au/sites/default/files/20160323-Bullying.pdf

31. 34% of doctors in training completing the Medical Training Survey in 2020 said they had experienced and/or witnessed bullying, harassment and/or discrimination at work. https://medicaltrainingsurvey.gov.au/News/Article/2020-medical-training-survey-results-are-now-available

32. Keltner, D. *The Power Paradox: How we gain and lose influence.* New York: Penguin Books, 2016.

33. Pfeffer, J. *Power: why some people have it - and others don't.* New York: Harper Collins, 2016.

34. Culture silences young doctors:

    CBC Radio 2 March 2018: https://www.cbc.ca/radio/whitecoat/metoo-in-medicine-1.4559561/metoo-in-medicine-culture-of-silence-keeps-med-students-from-reporting-abuse-by-their-mentors-1.4559570

    Four Corners Episode 25 May 2015: https://www.abc.net.au/4corners/at-their-mercy/6488010

35. Kadota, Yumiko. *Emotional Female.* Sydney: Penguin, 2021

36. Williamson AM, Feyer A. "Moderate sleep deprivation produces impairments in cognitive and motor performance equivalent to legally prescribed levels of alcohol intoxication." *Occupational and Environmental Medicine (*2000): 57:649-655. https://oem.bmj.com/content/57/10/649

37. Tawfik, DS, et al. (2018) "Physician Burnout, Well-being, and Work Unit Safety Grades in Relationship to Reported Medical Errors." Mayo Clin Proc. https://doi.org/10.1016/j.mayocp.2018.05.014 (Published online: July 09, 2018).

38. Dr Andrew Bryant died in 2017 from suicide. His wife, Susan bryant and their children published a letter about the months beforehand. https://www.brisbanetimes.com.au/national/queensland/i-didnt-see-it-coming-wife-of-brisbane-doctor-writes-letter-about-his-suicide-20170511-gw2ef2.html

    Dr Tasha Port died of suicide in 2020. Her parents Indrani and Graeme participated in the Crazy Socks 4 Docs panel discussion in 2021 pleading for change to working conditions for training doctors. https://www.crazysocks4docs.com.au/crazysocks4docs-day/crazysocks4docs-day-2021/crazysocks4docs-day-2021-video/

    Dr Chloe Abbott died of suicide in 2017. Her sister Micaela Abbott told the Australian Medical Students' Association (AMSA) it was due to systems failure not her sister's lack of resilience. https://www.smh.com.au/healthcare/she-was-eaten-alive-dr-chloe-abbotts-sister-micaelas-message-for-the-next-generation-of-doctors-20170704-gx4jt3.html

    There are thousands of these tragic stories. Families and friends of doctors imploring us to do better, to take better care of their loved ones.

39. Beyond Blue *National Mental Health Survey of Doctors and Medical Students* Australia 2013, updated in 2019. https://www.beyondblue.org.au/docs/default-source/research-project-files/bl1132-report—nmhdmss-full-report_web

40. R. Case, et. al. "Suicide prevention in High Risk Occupations: An evidence check rapid review The Sax Institute." NSW Ministry of Health 2020. https://www.monash.edu/medicine/news/latest/2020-articles/monash-university-report-identifies-occupations-with-greater-risk-of-suicide

41. https://www.beyondblue.org.au/docs/default-source/research-project-files/bl1132-report—nmhdmss-full-report_web

    G. Dawnay *Doctor suicide – how many more? BMJ Opinion June 13 2019.* https://blogs.bmj.com/bmj/2019/06/13/giles-dawnay-doctor-suicide-how-many-more/

    P. Anderson *Doctors' suicide rate highest of any profession* WebMed, Medscape Medical News 2018. https://www.webmd.com/mental-health/news/20180508/doctors-suicide-rate-highest-of-any-profession

42. Myers, M.F. *Why Physicians Die By Suicide.* New York: Springer, 2017.

## Chapter 2

43. World Health Organisation Constitiution, Definition of Health. https://www.who.int/about/governance/constitution

44. Seligman, M. *Flourish.* Sydney: Random House, 2011.

45. *F.A. Huppert and T.T.C.* "So Flourishing Across Europe: Application of a New Conceptual Framework for Defining Well-Being." *Social Indicators Research* (2011,2013): 110(3): 837–861.

46. *Open access online:* 10.1007/s11205-011-9966-7

47. PERMA – Positive emotions, Engagement, Relationships, Meaning, Accomplishment

48. The wellbeing Continuum is my adaptation of various other continuums, including that proposed by Gordon Allport in 1937. Allport considered mental illness and mental health as the two poles of a linear continuum. He described optimum functioning at the well end as having zeal about a number of interests and an ability to pursue them, an ability to accomplish daily responsibilities like self-care and insight into the external and internal worlds. https://positivepsychology.com/mental-health-continuum-model/

    Canada's The Working Mind mental health model is another example of a continuum of mental health – ill-injured-reacting-healthy. https://theworkimgmind.ca/continuum-self-check

49. Keyes, C.L.M. "The mental health continuum: from languishing to flourishing in life." *Journal of Health Social Behaviour* (2002): 43(2):207-22.

50. Segal, Leonie, Claire Marsh and Rob Heyes. "The real cost of training health professionals in Australia: it costs as much to build a dietician workforce as a dental workforce." J Health Serv Res Policy (2017): 22(2): 91–98. https://www.ncbi.nlm.nih.gov/pmc/articles/PMC5347354/

51. Allan, James, MD. "The Total Cost To Train a Physician." The Hospital Medical Director Blog. https://hospitalmedicaldirector.com/the-total-cost-to-train-a-physician/ (Accessed July 11, 2019.)

52. R. Davidson, Wellbeing is a skill presentation at Wisdom 2.0 - 31 March 2015. https://www.youtube.com/watch?v=EPGJU7W0N0I

53. The Links between the Dalai Lama and Neuroscience, NPR Nov 11 2005. https://www.npr.org/templates/story/story.php?storyId=5008565

54. Davidson, R. with S Begley. *The Emotional Life of the Brain.* Great Britain: Hodder and Stoughton, 2012.

55. Richie Davidson's wellbeing website and App can be found here: https://center-healthyminds.org

56. Matthew A. Killingsworth* and Daniel T. Gilbert, Science , 12 Nov 2010 Vol 330. https://wjh-www.harvard.edu/~dtg/KILLINGSWORTH%20&%20GILBERT%20(2010).pdf

57. Clark, T.R. *The 4 Stages of Psychological Safety – Defining the Path to Inclusion and Innovation.* California: Berrett-Koehler Publishers, Inc., 2020.

58. You can learn a lot more about psychological safety from Amy Edmondson too in her book A Fearless Organisation, 2018 John Wiley and Sons and here in this video https://www.youtube.com/watch?v=x9UwwY3xiiQ

59. Pfeffer, J. *Power: why some people have it - and others don't.* New York: Harper Collins, 2016. p9 and p236

60. M. Lerner and L. Montada (Editors). *Responses to Victimizations and Belief in a Just World.* New York: Plenum Press, 1998. https://link.springer.com/content/pdf/10.1007%2F978-1-4757-6418-5_1.pdf

## Chapter 3

61. https://www.sleephealthfoundation.org.au/pdfs/Special_Reports/SHF_Insomnia_Report_2019_Final_SHFlogo.pdf

62. National Sleep Foundation's sleep time duration recommendations: methodology and results summary 2015 Mar;1(1):40-43. https://pubmed.ncbi.nlm.nih.gov/29073412/

63. Matthew Walker, *Why We Sleep, Scribner, 2017*

64. One example of this was given by Dr Olivia Ong at her book launch on 9 Sept 2021 when she described wishing she had a catheter as a registrar so she wouldn't have to stop work to go to the bathroom.

65. Frankl, V.E. *Man's Search For Meaning.* Beacon Press, 1946

66. The phrase Default Mode Network was first used in 2001 by neurologist Marcus E. Raichle, around 2007 neuroscientists started using the term more and research increased exponentially and continues, there is not agreement across scientists. Here is a recent study describing some of what the Default Network might be doing. Gordon, EM, et. al. "Default-mode network streams for coupling to language and control systems." *PNAS* (2020): 117(29) 17308 – 17319. https://www.pnas.org/content/117/29/17308

67. Habits - a repeat performance. Neal, DT. Wood, W and Quinn, JM 2006. https://journals.sagepub.com/doi/10.1111/j.1467-8721.2006.00435.x

68. Duhigg, C. *The Power of Habit.* London: William Heinemann, 2020

69. Phillippa Lally, et. al. "How are habits formed: Modelling habit formation in the real world." *European Journal of Social Psychology* (2010): 40, 998–1009. http://repositorio.ispa.pt/bitstream/10400.12/3364/1/IJSP_998-1009.pdf

70. Mindfulness reduces stress:

    Martín-Asuero, A., and G. García-Banda. "The Mindfulness-Based Stress Reduction Program (MBSR) Reduces Stress-Related Psychological Distress in Healthcare Professionals." *The Spanish Journal of Psychology* 2010: *13*(2), 897-905. doi:10.1017/S1138741600002547

Chin, B., Slutsky, *et al.* "Mindfulness Training Reduces Stress at Work: a Randomized Controlled Trial." *Mindfulness* 2019: 10, 627–638. https://doi.org/10.1007/s12671-018-1022-0

Epstein, R. MD. *Attending, Medicine, Mindfulness and Humanity.* New York: Scribner, 2017

Germer, C and K. Neff. *Teaching the Mindful Self-Compassion Program.* New York: The Guilford Press, 2019.

Gilbert, P. and Choden. *Mindful Compassion.* Great Britain: Robinson, 2013.

Gilbert, P. *Living Like Crazy.* Great Britain: Annwyn House, 2017.

Hougaard, R., J. Carter and G. Coutts. *One Second Ahead.* Hampshire UK: Palgrave McMillan, 2016.

Hougaard, R and J. Carter. *The Mind of the Leader.* Boston: Harvard Business Review Press, 2018.

Rodski, S. *The Neuroscience of Mindfulness.* Sydney: Harper Collins Publishers, 2019.

71.  Langer, E. *Mindfulness.* Hatchette Books, 1989.

72.  Tusso, M.A., D.M. Santarelli and D. O'Rourke. "The Physiological effects of slow breathing in the healthy human." *Breathe (Sheff)* 2017: 13(4): 298–309. https://www.ncbi.nlm.nih.gov/pmc/articles/PMC5709795/

Nestor, J. *Breathe, The New Science of a Lost Art.* Penguin Life, 2021.

Johnson, W. *Breathing Through the Whole Body, Inner Traditions.* Vermont, 2012.

73.  Armstrong, K. Interoception: How We Understand Our Body's Inner Sensations, September 25, 2019. https://www.psychologicalscience.org/observer/interoception-how-we-understand-our-bodys-inner-sensations

Butley, DS and L. Moseley. *Explain Pain- A Clinician's Guide.* Adelaid: Noi Publications, 2017.

74.  Emotional literacy:

David, S. *Emotional Agility.* Great Britain: Penguin, 2016.

Goleman, D. *Emotional Intelligence* Great Britain Bloomsbury 1995

75.  Stoics value.... Stoics: https://onlinelibrary.wiley.com/doi/full/10.1111/acem.13967

76.  Salovey, P. and J.D. Mayer. "Emotional intelligence." *Imagination, Cognition, and Personality* 1990: *9,* 185–211.

77.  Research to say better accuracy with own emotions = more accuracy with others. Caruso, DR and Salovey, P. *The Emotionally Intelligent Manager* Josse-Bass, San Francisco, 2004

78.  Suppression

https://greatergood.berkeley.edu/article/item/how_to_regulate_your_emotions_without_suppressing_them

79. Duffy, B. *The Perils of Perception* Atlantic Books London 2018. See note #70 re: mindfulness

80. Hogg, Michael A. "Chapter 5 Social Identity Theory". *Contemporary Social Psychological Theories: Second Edition*, edited by Peter J. Burke. Redwood City: Stanford University Press, 2018, pp. 112-138. https://doi.org/10.1515/9781503605626-007

81. Lieberman, M.D. Social – Why Our Brains are Wired to Connect, Crown, 2013

82. Definitions of various biases. https://www.catalyst.org/2020/01/02/interrupt-unconscious-bias/

83. Hoffman, K.M., et. al. "Black people receiving pain relief. Racial bias in pain assessment and treatment recommendations, and false beliefs about biological differences between blacks and whites." *Proceedings of the National Academy of Sciences* 2016: 113(16): 4296-4301 doi:10.1073/pnas.1516047113

    Mathur, V.A., et. al. "Racial bias in pain perception and response: experimental examination of automatic and deliberate processes." *Journal of Pain* 2014: 15(5): 476-484. doi: 10.1016/j.jpain.2014.01.488

## Chapter 4

84. Shanafelt TD, et al. "Career fit and burnout among academic faculty." *Arch Intern Med* 2009: 169(10): 990-995.

    Shanafelt, Tait D., M.D. and John H. Noseworthy, M.D., CEO. "Executive Leadership and Physician Well-being: Nine Organizational Strategies to Promote Engagement and Reduce Burnout." *Mayo Clinic Proceedings* 2017: 92(1):129-146 http://dx.doi.org/10.1016/j.mayocp.2016.10.004 www.mayoclinicproceedings.org

85. Christine Sinsky MD Vice President, Professional Satisfaction AMA and Internist in Private Practice discusses the impact of leadership and 20% of doing what gives you joy at work for the Research Medical Library at University of Texas MD Anderson Cancer Center, 25-27 September 2017. https://www.youtube.com/watch?v=_A4h6A2p564

86. The idea of a dominant story or narrative is used extensively in Narrative Therapy founded by Michael White and Acceptance Commitment Therapy established by Steven C. Hayes.

    https://dulwichcentre.com.au/what-is-narrative-therapy/

    https://stevenchayes.com/category/acceptance-and-commitment-therapy/

    Russell Harris is one of the leading voices in Acceptance Commitment Therapy in Australia. There are lots of useful free resources on his site here: https://www.actmindfully.com.au/free-stuff/free-videos/

87. Michael B. Beverland, Francis J. Farrelly, The Quest for Authenticity in Consumption: Consumers' Purposive Choice of Authentic Cues to Shape Experienced Outcomes, *Journal of Consumer Research*, Volume 36, Issue 5, February 2010, Pages 838–856, https://doi.org/10.1086/615047

88. Rosanna K. Smith, George E. Newman, Ravi Dhar, Closer to the Creator: Temporal Contagion Explains the Preference for Earlier Serial Numbers, *Journal of Consumer Research*, Volume 42, Issue 5, February 2016, Pages 653–668, https://doi.org/10.1093/jcr/ucv054

89. Clear, J. *Atomic Habits*. Penguin London 2018

90. Hayes, S. *A Liberated Mind* Penguin 2019

91. Teo K, Lear S, Islam S, Mony P, Dehghan M, Li W, Rosengren A, Lopez-Jaramillo P, Diaz R, Oliveira G, Miskan M, Rangarajan S, Iqbal R, Ilow R, Puone T, Bahonar A, Gulec S, Darwish EA, Lanas F, Vijaykumar K, Rahman O, Chifamba J, Hou Y, Li N, Yusuf S; PURE Investigators. Prevalence of a healthy lifestyle among individuals with cardiovascular disease in high-, middle- and low-income countries: The Prospective Urban Rural Epidemiology (PURE) study. JAMA. 2013 Apr 17;309(15):1613-21. doi: 10.1001/jama.2013.3519. PMID: 23592106.

92. I first thought about role theory in relation to coaching and doctor well-being when I began my Coach training in 2017 at the Institute of Executive Coaching and Leadership when John Matthews and Jane Porter made it come alive in real time. I recommend the course highly to you if you are seeking to learn to work as an organisational Coach.

    Role Theory: http://psychology.iresearchnet.com/social-psychology/social-psychology-theories/role-theory/

## Chapter 5

93. Mick Fanning attacked by shark, https://www.youtube.com/watch?v=M6i0os6u0M0

94. Mick Fanning makes documentary about saving sharks. https://www.savethis-shark.com

95. Keller, A., Litzelman, K., Wisk, L. E., Maddox, T., Cheng, E. R., Creswell, P. D., & Witt, W. P. (2012). Does the perception that stress affects health matter? The association with health and mortality. *Health psychology : official journal of the Division of Health Psychology, American Psychological Association*, 31(5), 677–684. https://doi.org/10.1037/a0026743

96. The relation of strength of stimulus to rapidity of habit-formation. Robert M. Yerkes,John D. Dodson, 1908 Wiley Online Library. https://onlinelibrary.wiley.com/doi/10.1002/cne.920180503

97.	I first learnt about the red and green zone way of describing the stress and relaxation response from Paul Bedson at the Yarra Valley Learning and Living Centre on a meditation retreat in 2008.

98.	Hanson, R *Resilient*, Penguin, 2018

99.	Benson, H. MD with Klipper, M.Z. *The Relaxation Response* 1975 HarperTorch

100.	Horn, A.B. and Maercker, A. Intra and interpersonal emotion regulations and adjustment symptoms in couples: The role of co-brooding and co-reappraisal. BMC Psychology 4, 51 (2016) https://doi.org/10.1186/s40359-016-0159-7

101.	The quote *Suffering is optional* has been attribute to the Dalai Lama, Haruki Murakami, and M. Kathleen Casey. I learnt this equation from Rasmus Hougaard the Founder of the Potential Project. I have been associated with the Potential Project since 2014 teaching mindfulness and compassion skills to people in organisations including health, military, education and corporate. Many doctors have told me they have shared this equation with their patients and have found it helpful.

102.	See note 85 regarding 20% activities that you enjoy being the baseline.

103.	Germer, C and Neff, K. *Teaching the Mindful Self-Compassion Program,* The Guilford Press, NY, 2019

	Germer and Neff describe three elements of self compassion – Mindfulness, Common Humanity and Kindness.

104.	Self-Compassion Soothes the Savage EGO-Threat System: Effects on Negative Affect, Shame, Rumination, and Depressive Symptoms November 2013 Journal of Social and Clinical Psychology 2013(32):939-963

105.	Refer to notes 61-63 (sleep)

106.	https://www.prevention.com/health/sleep-energy/a20440036/napping-on-the-job-increases-productivity/

107.	Covey, S.R. *7 Habits of Highly Effective People* Simon Schuster 1989

108.	https://www.hush.org.au/

109.	Gratitude: https://greatergood.berkeley.edu/article/item/how_gratitude_changes_you_and_your_brain

110.	van Cuylenburg, H. *The Resilience Project, Finding Happiness Through Gratitude, Empathy and Mindfuness*, Random House Australia, 2019


## Chapter 6

111.	Y. Kadota, *Emotional Female,* Viking (Penguin), 2021, p320

112.	J.E. Groopman, How Doctors Think, Houghton Mifflin Company Boston 2008

113. Refer also notes 74, 76, 77.

https://langleygroup.com.au/whitepaper-emotional-intelligence-at-work/

114. David, S. *Emotional Agility* Penguin Great Britain 2016

115. Ekman, P. https://www.paulekman.com/blog/universality-of-emotions/

116. Atlas of Emotions, a dialogue between Paul Ekman and the Dalai Lama. http://atlasofemotions.org/#introduction/

117. Fredrickson B. L. (2001). The role of positive emotions in positive psychology. The broaden-and-build theory of positive emotions. *The American psychologist, 56*(3), 218–226. https://doi.org/10.1037//0003-066x.56.3.218

118. Feldman-Barrett, L. Emotions are Real. Emotion © 2012 American Psychological Association 2012, Vol. 12, No. 3, 413– 429. https://www.affective-science.org/pubs/2012/emotions-are-real.pdf

119. This snake story is real. It happened to my friend when she was out running in the Summer of 2020

120. Feldman-Barrett, L. *Seven and a Half Lessons About the Brain,* Marriner Books, 2020

121. Feldman-Barrett, L, Ted Talk – You aren't at the mercy of your emotions – your brain creates them. https://www.ted.com/talks/lisa_feldman_barrett_you_aren_t_at_the_mercy_of_your_emotions_your_brain_creates_them

122. Stickiness

Goleman, D and Davidson, RJ *Altered Traits, Science Reveals How Meditation Changes Your Mind, Brain and Body. New York*, Avery, 2018, p162

123. Vyjeyanthi S. Periyakoil, M.D.

Using metaphors in medicine Stanford School of Medicine. https://palliative.stanford.edu/pioneers-in-palliative-care/dr-porter-storey/dr-periyakoil-using-metaphors-in-medicine/

124. Zak, PJ The neuroscience of trust, HBR Jan-Feb 2017 p84-90. https://hbr.org/2017/01/the-neuroscience-of-trust

125. Google's Project Aristotle, high trust teams share emotions and become more effective. https://rework.withgoogle.com/print/guides/5721312655835136/

126. Brown, B. *Daring Greatly,* Penguin, London, 2016

127. Brown, B. *Dare to Lead,* Vermilion, London, 2018

128. Recalibrate is our Immersion Doctor Care Program. We work in closed small groups with doctors for 6 -10 months combining individual coaching and small group work to build intra and interpersonal skill. Including – mindfulness, emotional intelligence, communication, leadership, preventing burnout.

129. I learnt this Kindness activity from Lorraine Dickey MD at The Gathering of Kindness in 2018. Lorraine founded The Narrative Initiative in Pennsylvania in 2017.

130. Doctors being told they are weak or reading the social norm as such:
   - onthewards.org blog, 18 April 2015, Call me if you need me. But remember- it's a sign of weakness.
   - Multiple speakers at Ending Physician Burnout Global Summit August 2021.
   - Many of the doctors I have worked with as coach have stories of supervisors telling them they are perhaps too weak of mind or fortitude to be a doctor. Almost all have stories of this being an all pervading social norm of medicine – that if you fail or ask for help, which is regarded as akin to failing, you are too weak to be a doctor anyway...
   - Wilson, H. and Cunningham, W. *Being a Doctor – Understanding Medical Practice.* 2014 Royal College of General Practitioners UK

131. Susan David says Courage is fear walking. Brene Brown says resilient people embrace vulnerability maintaining their sense of worth and wholeheartedness. She goes on to describe vulnerability as "the birth place of innovation, creativity and change"

132. Evolution theory of shame

133. Cross-cultural invariances in the architecture of shame

Daniel Sznycer, Dimitris Xygalatas, Elizabeth Agey, Sarah Alami, Xiao-Fen An, Kristina I. Ananyeva, Quentin D. Atkinson, Bernardo R. Broitman, Thomas J. Conte, Carola Flores, Shintaro Fukushima, Hidefumi Hitokoto, Alexander N. Kharitonov, Charity N. Onyishi, Ike E. Onyishi, Pedro P. Romero, Joshua M. Schrock, J. Josh Snodgrass, Lawrence S. Sugiyama, Kosuke Takemura, Cathryn Townsend, Jin-Ying Zhuang, C. Athena Aktipis, Lee Cronk, Leda Cosmides, John Tooby

Proceedings of the National Academy of Sciences Sep 2018, 115 (39) 9702-9707; DOI: 10.1073/pnas.1805016115. https://www.pnas.org/content/115/39/9702

134. Brown, B Ted Talk *Listening to Shame 2012* http://www.ted.com/talks/brene_brown_listening_to_shame/up-next?language=en

135. Neff, K. *Fierce Self- Compassion*, Penguin UK, 2021

## Chapter 7

136. Sofer, OJ. *Say What Your Mean.* Shambala Publications. Colorado 2018 *p21*

137. Multitasking:

Multitasking Splits the Brain

The brain divides and conquers so that we can perform two tasks at once—but there are limits Gisela Telis 15 April 2010. https://www.science.org/content/article/multitasking-splits-brain

American Psychological Association Multitasking: Switching costs March 2006. https://www.apa.org/research/action/multitask

Susan Weinschenk Ph.D.Psychology Today 18 Sept 2012. https://www.psychology-today.com/au/blog/brain-wise/201209/the-true-cost-multi-tasking

138. No time for compassion

Riess, H, Kelley, J. Bailey RW, Dunn, EJ and Phillips, M. Empathy Training for Resident Physicians: A Randomized Control Trial of a Neuroscience-Informed Curriculum. J of General Internal Medicine 27, 10 (October 2021)1280-6

139. Fogarty, LA, Curbow, BA, Wingard, JR, McDonnell, K and Somerfield, MR. *Can 40 Seconds of Compassion Reduce Patient Anxiety?* J of Clinical Oncology 17, 1 (January 1999): 371-9

140. Bylund, CL and Makoul, G. *Examining Empathy in Medical Encounters: An Observational Study Using the Empathic Communication Coding System.* Health Communication 18 n2 2005: 123-40

141. Youngson, R. *Time to Care.* Rebelheart Publishers 2012

142. Compassion writers

Bloom, P. *Against Empathy* Harper Collins Publishers, New York 2016

Epstein, R. MD *Attending, Medicine, Mindfulness and Humanity* . Scribner 2017 New York

Halpern, J. *From Detached Concern to Empathy, Humanizing Medical Practice.* Oxford University Press new York 2001

Trzeciak, S and Mazzarelli, A. *Compassionomics, The Revolutionary Scientific Evidence That Caring Makes a Difference.* Studer Group, Florida 2019

143. Compassion: a scoping review of the healthcare literature

Shane Sinclair, Jill M. Norris, Shelagh J. McConnell, Harvey Max Chochinov, Thomas F. Hack, Neil A. Hagen,Susan McClement, and Shelley Raffin Bouchal, BMC Palliat Care. 2016; 15: 6, Published online 19 Jan 2016. doi: 10.1186/s12904-016-0080-0. https://www.ncbi.nlm.nih.gov/pmc/articles/PMC4717626/

144. Kindness is contagious

Klaber , RE. *Kindness: an underrated currency*

BMJ 2019; 367 doi: https://doi.org/10.1136/bmj.l6099 (Published 16 December 2019)Cite this as: BMJ 2019;367:l6099

Tang, W., Wu, D., Yang, F. *et al.* How kindness can be contagious in healthcare. *Nature Med* 27, 1142–1144 (2021). https://doi.org/10.1038/s41591-021-01401-x. https://www.nature.com/articles/s41591-021-01401-x

Mental Health Foundation, UK. Kindness Research Briefing (Scotland). https://www.mentalhealth.org.uk/campaigns/mental-health-awareness-week/scotland-kindness-research

Kelly, J.D. Your Best Life: Kindness is Its Own Reward. *Clin Orthop Relat Res* 474, 1775–1777 (2016). https://doi.org/10.1007/s11999-016-4927-8. https://link.springer.com/article/10.1007/s11999-016-4927-8

145. Singh Ospina N, Phillips KA, Rodriguez-Gutierrez R, Castaneda-Guarderas A, Gionfriddo MR, Branda ME, Montori VM. Eliciting the Patient's Agenda- Secondary Analysis of Recorded Clinical Encounters. J Gen Intern Med. 2019 Jan;34(1):36-40. doi: 10.1007/s11606-018-4540-5. Epub 2018 Jul 2. PMID: 29968051; PMCID: PMC6318197.

Phillips, K.A., Ospina, N.S. & Montori, V.M. Physicians Interrupting Patients. *J GEN INTERN MED* 34, 1965 (2019). https://doi.org/10.1007/s11606-019-05247-5

Phillips KA, Ospina NS. Physicians Interrupting Patients. *JAMA.* 2017;318(1):93–94. doi:10.1001/jama.2017.6493

146. Mogilner, C. Chance, Z and Norton, MI. *Giving Time Gives You Time* Psychological Science 23 n10 (1 October 2012): 1233-8

147. *I've learned that people will forget what you said, people will forget what you did, but people will never forget how you made them feel,* American Poet Maya Angelou

148. Keltner, D *The Power Paradox, How we gain and lose influence.* Penguin UK 2017

149. Trimbolli, O. *Deep Listening, Impact Beyond Words. Oscar Trimbolli Sydney 2017*

150. Mehrabian, A., & Ferris, S. R. (1967). Inference of attitudes from nonverbal communication in two channels. *Journal of Consulting Psychology, 31*(3), 248–252. https://doi.org/10.1037/h0024648

151. Hojat M, Mangione S, Nasca TJ, Rattner S, Erdmann JB, Gonnella JS, Magee M. An empirical study of decline in empathy in medical school. Med Educ. 2004 Sep;38(9):934-41. doi: 10.1111/j.1365-2929.2004.01911.x. PMID: 15327674.

Neumann M, Edelhäuser F, Tauschel D, Fischer MR, Wirtz M, Woopen C, Haramati A, Scheffer C. Empathy decline and its reasons: a systematic review of studies with medical students and residents. Acad Med. 2011 Aug;86(8):996-1009. doi: 10.1097/ACM.0b013e318221e615. PMID: 21670661.

Hojat, Mohammadreza PhD; Shannon, Stephen C. DO; DeSantis, Jennifer MEd; Speicher, Mark R. PhD, MHA; Bragan, Lynn; Calabrese, Leonard H. DO Does Empathy Decline in the Clinical Phase of Medical Education? A Nationwide, Multi-Institutional, Cross-Sectional Study of Students at DO-Granting Medical Schools, Academic Medicine: June 2020 - Volume 95 - Issue 6 - p 911-918. doi: 10.1097/ACM.0000000000003175

152. Definition of empathy from Oren Jay Sofer p103 (see note 135)

153. O'Brien, C. *Never Say Die,* Harper Collins Publishers, Australia, 2008

O'Brien, J. *This is Gail, Life with and after Chris O'Brien* Harper Collins Publishers Australia 2016

154. Singer T, Seymour B, O'Doherty J, Kaube H, Dolan RJ, Frith CD. Empathy for pain involves the affective but not sensory components of pain. Science. 2004 Feb 20;303(5661):1157-62. doi: 10.1126/science.1093535. PMID: 14976305.

The Journal of Cognitive Neuro Science interview with Tania Singer 2013. https://www.cogneurosociety.org/empathy_pain/

Tania Singer, The Neuroscience of Compassion, 9 March 2015, World Economic Forum. https://www.youtube.com/watch?v=n-hKS4rucTY

155. Halpern, J. *From Detached Concern to Empathy, Humanizing Medical Practice.* Oxford University Press New York 2001

156. Esch, T., & Stefano, G. B. (2011). The neurobiological link between compassion and love. *Medical science monitor : international medical journal of experimental and clinical research, 17*(3), RA65–RA75. https://doi.org/10.12659/msm.881441

157. The Oxford Handbook of Compassion Science. Edited by Emma M. Seppälä, Emiliana Simon-Thomas, Stephanie L. Brown, Monica C. Worline, C. Daryl Cameron, and James R. Doty Oxford University Press USA 2017

158. Dowling T. (2018). Compassion does not fatigue!. *The Canadian veterinary journal 59*(7), 749–750.

Contesting the term 'compassion fatigue': Integrating findings from social neuroscience and self-care research, Anne Hofmeyer, Kate Kennedy, Ruth Taylor, Science Direct Collegian, Volume 27, Issue 2, April 2020, Pages 232-237. https://reader.elsevier.com/reader/sd/pii/S1322769619301672?token=A4A5F18455F34D5E5C35307822FF7A2A1C8C60B6AB20F6F0A2587BBE8B9FF71107FCEA18FF3368B011EE477D8CEB2111&originRegion=us-east-1&originCreation=20211004014451

159. K-ISBAR

Adding kindness at handover to improve our collegiality: the K-ISBAR tool

David J Brewster and Bruce P Waxman. Med J Aust 2018; 209 (11): . || doi: 10.5694/mja18.00755
Published online: 10 December 2018. https://www.mja.com.au/system/files/issues/209_11/10.5694mja18.00755.pdf

## Chapter 8

160. M. Seligman, Flourish Random House, Sydney 2011

161. WHO *Mental health: strengthening our response* 30 March 2018. https://www.who.int/news-room/fact-sheets/detail/mental-health-strengthening-our-response

162. Social isolation, loneliness, and mortality

Andrew Steptoe, Aparna Shankar, Panayotes Demakakos, Jane Wardle

Proceedings of the National Academy of Sciences Apr 2013, 110 (15) 5797-5801; DOI:10.1073/pnas.1219686110. https://www.pnas.org/content/110/15/5797.full

163. Yeginsu, Ceylan. UK Appoints a Minister for Loneliness. *New York Times*, January 17, 2018

164. J. Abbott, M Lim, R Eres, K Long and R. Mathews *The impact of loneliness on the health and wellbeing of Australians* Australian Psychological Society InPsych 2018, v40 issue6. https://www.psychology.org.au/for-members/publications/inpsych/2018/December-Issue-6/The-impact-of-loneliness-on-the-health-and-wellbei

165. 300th of a second to decide who to trust.

Amygdala Responsivity to High-Level Social Information from Unseen Faces Jonathan B. Freeman, Ryan M. Stolier, Zachary A. Ingbretsen and Eric A. Hehman Journal of Neuroscience 6 August 2014, 34 (32) 10573-10581; DOI: https://doi.org/10.1523/JNEUROSCI.5063-13.2014

166. Harvard Longitudinal Study. Good genes are nice, but joy is better. The Harvard Gazette. Liz Mineo 11 April 2017. https://news.harvard.edu/gazette/story/2017/04/over-nearly-80-years-harvard-study-has-been-showing-how-to-live-a-healthy-and-happy-life/

167. Holt-Lunstad J, Smith TB, Baker M, Harris T, Stephenson D. Loneliness and social isolation as risk factors for mortality: a meta-analytic review. Perspect Psychol Sci. 2015 Mar;10(2):227-37. doi: 10.1177/1745691614568352. PMID: 25910392.

168. John Cocioppa, in *Lost Connections by Johann Hari, Bloomsbury, Great Britain, 2019, p78*

169. Gallup best friends

https://www.gallup.com/workplace/237530/item-best-friend-work.aspx

https://www.gallup.com/workplace/236213/why-need-best-friends-work.aspx

170. Women in the healthcare workforce

Australian Institute of Health and Welfare Report 2018. https://www.aihw.gov.au/getmedia/c4d58e5e-c721-4dbe-8ed8-969afbcfdd3e/aihw-aus-221-chapter-2-3.pdf.aspx

OECD numbers: https://www.oecd.org/gender/data/women-make-up-most-of-the-health-sector-workers-but-they-are-under-represented-in-high-skilled-jobs.htm

171. Doctors do not speak honestly with each other about their mental health - here is a selection of the many authors who have written about this. At the Ending Physician Burnout Global Summit 24-26 August 2021 many speakers told of their experience of this. My coaching clients tell me this every week. Some examples of doctors writing about the hidden nature of their mental health include:

Drummond, D. Stop Physician Burnout, Dike Drummond, 2014

Pearl, R. Uncaring, note #1

Youngson, R, note #141

Groopman, J, note #112

*Bernard, R and Cohen, S. *Physician Wellness, The Rock Star Doctor's Guide.* Published by authors 2018

*Wilson, H. *Being a Doctor* Royal College of General Practitioners, London 2014

*Lipsenthal, L. *Finding Balance in a Medical Life*, 2007 USA

*Simonds, GR and Sotile, WM *The Thriving Physician, How to Avoid Burnout by Choosing Resilience Throughout Your Medical Career*, Studer Group, 2019

172. America's Loneliest Workers, According to Research by S. Anchor, GR Kellerman, A Reece and A. Robichaux. March 19, 2018 HBR. https://hbr.org/2018/03/americas-loneliest-workers-according-to-research

173. S. Godin, *Tribes*, Portfolio Penguin, New York, 2008

174. Recalibrate is our Immersion Doctor Care Program, see note 128.

175. Francis J. Flynn and Vanessa K.B. Lake, If You Need Help, Just Ask: Underestimating Compliance With Direct Requests For Help. 2008 Vol 95, No 1, 128-143. Journal of Personality and Social Psychology. https://www.researchgate.net/publication/229176033_If_You_Need_Help_Just_Ask_Underestimating_Compliance_With_Direct_Requests_for_Help

176. 5 Ways to Decide Who You Can Trust. Before you commit, are you sure you're in your "wise mind"? Posted November 4, 2014 Psychology Today Melanie Greenberg. https://www.psychologytoday.com/au/blog/the-mindful-self-express/201411/5-ways-decide-who-you-can-trust

177. B. Ware, *Regrets of the Dying,* Hay House, 2019

**Chapter 9**

178. Robert Keegan, The Evolution of the Self. https://m.youtube.com/watch?v=bhRNMj6UNYY

179. Keegan, R. and Lahey, L. *Immunity to Change*

# FURTHER READING

As well as formal references, there are a lot of books and articles that inform my practice and this work. Some of them provide background understanding and others serve as inspiration provoking new thinking and inspiration. In case any of them are of interest or benefit to you, I have provided this further reading list.

**Change Your Brain, Change Your Life** by D.G. Amen
*Three Rivers Press, New York 1998*

**Mastering Leadership** by R.J. Anderson and W.A. Adams
*John Wiley and Sons, New Jersey 2016*

**The Plastic Mind** by S. Begley
*Constable and Robinson, London 2009*

**Physical Wellness: The rock star doctor's guide** by R. Bernard and S. Cohen
*Rebekah Bernard md and Steven Cohen PsyD, USA 2015*

**Games People Play: The psychology of human relationships** by E. Berne
*Penguin Books, USA 1964*

**Against Empathy: The case for rational compassion** by P. Bloom
*HarperCollins Publishers, New York 2016*

**Dancing at the River's Edge: A patient and her doctor negotiate life with chronic illness** by A. Brill and M.D. Lockshin
*Schaffner Press, Inc., Arizona 2009*

**Daring Greatly: How the courage to be vulnerable transforms the way we live, love, parent and lead** by B. Brown
*Penguin Books, London 2013*

**Dare to Lead** by B. Brown
*Vermilion, London 2018*

**The Coaching Habit** by M. Bungay Stanier
*Box of Crayons Press, Canada 2016*

**The Mindful Leader** by M. Bunting
*Wiley and Sons, Australia 2016*

**Shame** by J. Burgo
*St. Martin's Press, USA 2018*

**The Emotionally Intelligent Manager** by D.T. Caruso and P. Salovey
*Jossey-Bass, San Fransisco 2004*

**Clark, T.R. The 4 Stages of Psychological Safety: Defining the path to inclusion and innovation** by T.R. Clark
*Berrett-Koehler Publishers, California 2020*

**Atomic Habits: An easy and proven way to build good habits and break bad ones** by J. Clear
*Random House, USA 2018*

**From Good to Great** by J.C. Collins
*Random House, UK 2001*

**The Health Hazard: Take control, restore wellbeing and optimise impact** by A. Coughlan
*Grammar Factory Publishing, Canada 2021*

**The 7 Habits of Highly Effective People** by S.R. Covey
*Simon and Schuster, UK 1989*

**The Compete Handbook of Coaching 2nd Ed** by E. Cox, T. Bachkirova and D. Clutterbuck (Eds)
*Sage, London 2014*

**Flow: the psychology of optimal experience** by M. Csikszentmihalyl
*HarperCollins, New York 1990*

**Presence: Bringing your boldest self to your biggest challenges** by A. Cuddy
*Orion ,Great Britain 2016*

**Emotional Agility** by S. David
*Penguin Life, Great Britain 2016*

**The Polyvagal Theory in Therapy – Engaging the Rhythm of Regulation** by D. Dana
*W.W. Norton and Company, 2018*

**Davidson, R and Begley, S. The Emotional Life of Your Brain** by R. Davidson and S. Begley
*Hodder and Stoughton, Great Britain 2012*

**Mindful Medical Practice: Clinical narratives and therapeutic insights** by P. Dobkin (Ed)
*Springer, Switzerland 2015*

**Grit: Why passion and resilience are the secrets to success** by A. Duckworth

**Narrative Coaching – the definitive guide to bringing new stories to life 2nd Ed** by D.B. Drake
*CNC Press, California 2018*

**Stop Physician Burnout: What to do when working harder isn't working** by D. Drummond
*Dike Drummond, USA 2014*

**The Power of Habit: Why we do what we do and how to change** by C. Duhigg
*William Heinemann, London 2012*

**The Perils of Perception: Why we're wrong about nearly everything** by B. Duffy
*Atlantic Books, Great Britain 2018*

**Mindset: How you can fulfil your potential** by C.S. Dweck
*Constable and Robinson, London 2012*

**Biased: Uncovering the hidden prejudice that shapes what we see, think and do** by J.L. Eberhardt
*Penguin Books, US 2020*

**The Fearless Organisation** by A. Edmondson
*John Wiley and Sons, New Jersey 2019*

**Also Human: The Inner Lives of Doctors** by C. Elton
*Windmill Books London, 2018*

**Going on Being** by M. Epstein
*Wisdom Publications, Boston 2008*

**Attending: Medicine, Mindfulness and Humanity** by R. Epstein
*Scribner, New York 2017*

**Seven and a Half Lessons About the Brain** by L. Feldman Barett
*Picador, New York 2020*

**Remedy for Burnout: Prescriptions doctors use to find meaning in medicine** by S. Fitch
*Langdon Street Press Minneapolis, 2014*

**Tiny Habits: The small changes that change everything** by B.J. Fogg
*Virgin Books, London 2019*

**The Putting Patients First Field Guide: Global lessons in Designing and Implementing Patient-Centred Care** by S.B. Frampton, P.A. and S. Guastello
*Jossey-Bass, San Francisco 2013*

**Positivity: Discover the upward spiral that will change your life** by B.L. Fredrickson
*Harmony Books, New York 2009*

**Be Brilliant: How To Lead A Life of Influence** by J. Garner
*John Wiley and Sons, Australia Ltd 2020*

**Better: A surgeon's notes on performance** by A. Gawande
*Profile Books Ltd, London 2008*

**Beneath the White Coat: Doctors, their minds and mental health** by C. Gerada (Ed)
*Routledge, New York 2021*

**Teaching the Mindful Self-Compassion Program: A guide for professionals** by C. Germer and K. Neff
*The Guilford Press, New York 2019*

**Better Doctors, Better Patients, Better Decisions** by G. Gigerenzer and J.A. Muir Gray
*MIT Press, Massachusetts 2011*

**Mindful Compassion. Robinson** by P. Gilbert and Choden
*London 2013*

**Living Like Crazy** by P. Gilbert
*Annwyn House, Great Britain 2017*

**Tribes: We need you to lead us** by S. Godin
*Portfolio, New York 2008*

**Emotional Intelligence: Why it can matter more than IQ** by D. Goleman
*Bantam Books, US 1995*

**Focus: the hidden driver of excellence** by D. Goleman
*Bloomsbury, Great Britain 2014*

**A Force for Good: The Dalai Lama's vision for our world** by D. Goleman
*Bloomsbury Publishing, Great Britain 2015*

**Altered Traits: Science reveals how meditation changes your mind, brain and body** by D. Goleman and R.J. Davidson
*Avery, New York 2017*

**Grant, A. Think Again** by A. Grant
*WH Allen, London 2021*

**Mind Over Mood- Change how you feel** by changing the way you think by D. Greenberger and C.A. Padesky
*The Guilford Press, New York 1995*

**How Doctors Think** by J. Groopman
*Houghton Mifflin Company, New York 2007*

**Standing at the Edge: Finding freedom where fear and courage meet** by J. Halifax
*Flatiron Books, New York 2018*

**From Detached Concern to Empathy: Humanizing medical practice** by J. Halpern
*Oxford University Press, New York 2001*

**Buddha's Brain: the practical neuroscience of happiness, love and wisdom** by R. Hanson and R. Mendius
*New Harbinger Publications, California 2009*

**Resilient: Find Your Inner Strength** by R. Hanson
*Rider, London 2018*

**Neurodharma** by R. Hanson
*Rider, London 2020*

**Lost Connections: Uncovering the real causes of depression – and the unexpected solutions** by J. Hari
*Bloomsbury Circus, London 2018*

**The Complete Guide to a Good Night's Sleep** by C. Harrington
*Pan Macmillan, Australia 2014*

**A Liberated Mind: The essential guide to ACT** by S.C. Hayes
*Vermilion, London 2019*

**The Happiness Trap** by R. Harris
*Exisle Publishing, UK 2007*

**Mindful Learning** by C. Hassed and R. Chambers
*Shambala, Boston 2015*

**Wilful Blindness** by M. Heffernan
*Simon and Schuster, UK 2019*

**The Medicine: A Doctor's Notes** by K. Hitchcock
*Black Inc., Melbourne 2020*

**Evidence-Based Practice Across the Health Professions 2nd Ed** by T. Hoffman, S Bennett and C. Del Mar
*Elsevier, Australia 2013*

**The Obstacle is the Way** by R. Holiday
*Profile Books, London 2015*

**The Mind of the Leader** by R. Hougaard and J. Carter
*Harvard Business Review Press, Boston 2018*

**Burnout: Your first 10 steps** by A. Imms
*Amy Imms, Australia 2019*

**A Fearless Heart: Why compassion is the key to greater wellbeing** by T. Jinpa
*Penguin Group, USA 2015*

**Who Moved My Cheese** by S. Johnson
*Random House, UK 1999*

**Breathing Through The Whole Body** by W. Johnson
*Inner Traditions, Vermont 2012*

**Stress Less: proven methods to reduce stress, manage anxiety and lift your mood** by M. Johnstone and M. Player
*Pan Macmillan, Australia 2019*

**Coming To Our Senses** by J. Kabat-Zinn
*Hyperion, New York 2005*

**Full Catastrophe Living** by J. Kabat-Zinn
*Delta Trade Paperbacks, New York 2009*

**Emotional Female** by Y. Kadota
*Viking, Australia 2021*

**Power and Love: A theory and practice of social change** by A. Kahane
*Berrett-Koehler Publishers, California 2010*

**Thinking Fast and Slow** by D. Kahneman
*Penguin Books, London 2012*

**When Breath Becomes Air** by P. Kalanithi
*The Bodley Head, London 2016*

**Mindfulness, Acceptance, and Positive Psychology: The seven foundations of well-being** by T.B. Kashdan and J. Ciarrochi (Eds)
*Context Press, California 2013.*

**This is Going To Hurt** by A. Kay
*Pam Macmillan, UK 2018*

**Immunity To Change** by R. Kegan and L. Laskow Lahey
*Harvard Business Press, Boston 2009*

**An Everyone Culture** by R. Kegan and L. Laskow Lahey
*Harvard Business Review Press, Boston 2016*

**The Power Paradox: How we gain and lose influence** by D. Keltner
*Penguin Books USA, 2017*

**Finding Meaning: The sixth stage of grief** by D. Kessler
*Rider, London, 2019*

**That's Not How We Do It Here!** By J. Kotter and H. Rathgeber
*Portfolio Penguin, UK 2016*

**The Five Dysfunctions of a Team: a leadership fable** by P. Lencioni
*Jossey-Bass, California 2002*

**Know Yourself, Forget Yourself** by M. Lesser
*New World Library, California 2013*

**Lieberman, M.D. Social: Why our brains are wired to connect** by M.D. Lieberman
*Broadway Books, New York 2013*

**Finding Balance in a Medical Life** by L. Lipsenthal
*Finding Balance Inc., California 2007*

**Tribal Leadership: Leveraging natural groups to build a thriving organization** by D. Logan, J. King and H. Fischer-Wright
*Harper Business, New York 2008*

**Trust and Betrayal: Morality and the emotions in surgery** by D. Macintosh
*Australian Scholarly Publishing, Melbourne 2016*

**Good Leaders Ask Great Questions: Your foundation for successful leadership** by J.C. Maxwell
*Hatchett Book Group, New York 2014*

**Beyond the Stethoscope: Doctors' stories of reclaiming hope, heart and healing in medicine** by L. Mayes
*Heart Works Press, Australia 2017*

**Building Your Resilience: How to thrive in a challenging job** by K. McEwan
*Mindset Publications, South Australia 2016*

**The iRest Program for Healing PTSD** by R. Miller
*New Harbinger Publications, California 2015*

**Coaching Psychology Manual 2nd Ed.** By M. Moore, E. Jackson and B. Tschannin-Moran
*Wolters Kluwer, US 2016*

**Lead Like A Coach: How to get the most out of any team** by K. Morley
*Major Street Publishing, Melbourne 2018*

**You're Not Listening: What you're missing and why it matters** by K. Murphy
*Vintage, UK 2020*

**Cautionary Tales: Authentic Case Histories from Medical Practice 2nd Ed.** By J. Murtagh
*McGraw-Hill, Australia 2011*

**Burnout: The Secret to Unlocking the Stress Cycle** by E. Nagoski and A. Nagoski
*Ballantine Books, New York 2019*

**Fierce Self-Compassion** by K. Neff
*Penguin, UK 2021*

**Being Peace** by T. Nhat Hanh
*Parallax Press, Berkeley 2005*

**You Are Here: Discovering the Magic of the Present Moment** by T. Nhat Hanh
*Shambala, Boston 2009*

**Silver Linings: True stories of resilience from a general practice** by M. Nayagam
*Dr Mrin Nayagam, Australia 2017*

**Breath: The new science of a lost art** by J. Nestor
*Penguin Life, USA 2021*

**Mindfulness and Character Strengths: a practical guide to flourishing** by R.M. Niemiec
*Hogrefe Publishing, Boston 2013*

**Medicine and Compassion** by C. Nyima and D.R. Shlim
*Wisdom Publications, Boston 2015*

**Never Say Die** by C. O'Brien
*HarperCollins Publishers, Australia 2016*

**This is Gail** by J. O'Brien
*HarperCollins Publishers, 2016*

**Do One Thing Different: Ten Simple Ways to Change Your Life** by B. O'Hanlon
*Quill, New York 1999*

**Communication: Core interpersonal skills for Health Professionals 3rd Ed.** By G. O'Toole
*Elsevier, Australia 2017*

**Handbook of Coaching Psychology: a guide for practitioners 2nd Ed.** by S. Palmer and A. Whybrow
*Routledge, UK 2019*

**Leadership Embodiment: How the way we sit and stand can change the way we think and speak** by W. Palmer and J. Crawford
*Embodiment International, California 2013*

**Burnout: A guide to identifying burnout and pathways to recovery** by G. Parker, G. Tavella and K. Eyers
*Allen and Unwin, Sydney 2021*

**Uncaring: How the culture of medicine kills doctors and patients** by R. Pearl
*PublicAffairs, USA 2021*

**Power: Why Some People Have It - and Others Don't** by J. Pfeffer
*HarperCollins Publishers, New York 2010*

**The War of Art: Break Through the Blocks and Win Your Inner Creative Battles** by S. Pressfield
*Black Irish Entertainment LLC, New York 2012*

**Lean Forward Into Your Life** by M. Radmacher
*Conari Press, California 2007*

**The Leading Edge** by H. Ranson
*Viking, Australia 2021*

**Out of Our Minds: The Power of Being Creative 3rd Ed.** by K. Robinson
*John Wiley and Sons, UK 2017.*

**Coaching with the Brain in Mind** by D. Rock and L.J. Page
*John Wiley and Sons, New Jersey 2009*

**Rodski, S. The Neuroscience of Mindfulness** by S. Rodski
*Harper Collins Publishers, Australia 2017*

**Self-Care Revolution** by E. Rondina
*Ellen Rondina, California 2018*

**The Body Remembers** by B. Rothschild
*WW Norton and Company, New York 2000*

**Lean In: Women, work and the will to lead** by S. Sandberg
*WH Allen, London 2015*

**Behave: The biology of humans at our best and worst** by R. Sapolsky
*Vintage, London 2017*

**Radical Candor** by Kim Scott

**Emotions: An Owner's Manual** by J. Seldon
*Outskirts Press, USA 2017*

**Authentic Happiness** by M. Seligman
*Random House, Australia 2002*

**Flourish** by M. Seligman
*William Heinemann, Sydney 2011*

**The Fifth Discipline** by P.M. Senge
*Random House, Australia 1992*

**The Oxford Handbook of Compassion Science** by E.M. Seppala, E. Simon-Thomas, S. Brown, M.C. Worline, C.D. Cameron and J. Doty
*Oxford University Press, USA 2017*

**The Art and Science of Mindfulness** by S.L. Shapiro and L.E. Carlson
*American Psychological Association, Washington 2009*

**Coaching to the Human Soul: Ontological Coaching and Deep Change, Vol I (2003) and II (2007)**
*Alan Sieler Publishing Solutions P/L, Australia*

**Love, Medicine and Miracles** by B. Siegel
*Rider, UK 1999*

**The Mindful Brain** by D.J. Siegel
*W.W.Norton and Company, New York 2007*

**Mindsight: Change your brain and your life** by D.J. Siegel
*Scribe Publications, Melbourne 2009*

**The Developing Mind 2nd Ed.** by D.J. Siegel
*The Guilford Press, New York 2012*

**Presence-Based Leadership: complexity practices for clarity, resilience, and results that matter** by D. Silsbee
*Yes! Global, North Carolina 2018*

**Skills for Communication with Patients 3rd Ed** by J. Silvermann, S. Kurtz and J. Draper
*CRC Press, Florida 2013*

**The Thriving Physician** by G.R. Simonds and W.M. Sotile
*Studer Group, LLC, Florida 2018*

**The Infinite Game** by S. Sinek
*Penguin, US 2019*

**Say What You Mean: A mindful approach to nonviolent communication** by O.J. Sofer
*Shambala, Colorado 2018*

**What It Takes To Be A Doctor** by R. Srivastava
*Simon and Schuster, Australia 2018*

**In This Moment** by K.D. Strosahl and P.J. Robinson
*New Harbinger Publications, California 2015*

**The Well Gardened Mind** by S. Stuart-Smith
*William Collins, London 2020*

**The Advantage of Being Useless: The Tao and the Counsellor** by G. Sweet
*The Dunmoor Press, New Zealand 1989*

**Joy on Demand: The art of discovering the happiness within** by C.M. Tan
*HarperCollins Publishers, New York 2016*

**Deep Listening: Impact beyond words** by O. Trimboli
*Oscar Trimboli, Australia, 2017*

**Compassionomics: The Revolutionary Scientific Evidence That Caring Makes A Difference** by S. Trzeciak and A. Mazzarelli
*Studer Group, Florida 2019*

**The Body Keeps the Score** by B. Vander Kolk
*Penguin Books, New York 2015*

**It Takes Five To Tango: From Competition to Cooperation in Health Care** by V. Voelter
*Macmillan, US 2021*

**Why We Sleep: The new science of sleep and dreams** by M. Walker
*Penguin Books, USA 2017*

**How We Work** by L. Weiss
*HarperCollins, New York 2019*

**Integral Meditation** by K. Wilber
*Shambala, Colorado 2016*

**Caste: The Lies That Divide Us** by I. Wilkerson
*Allen Lane, US 2020*

**Mindfulness: a practical guide to finding peace in a frantic world** by M. Williams and D. Penman
*Piatkus, Great Britain 2012*

**Being A Doctor: Understanding medical practice** by H. Wilson and W. Cunningham
*Royal College of General Practitioners, UK 2014.*

**Redirect: Changing the stories we live by,** by T.D. Wilson
*Penguin Books, London 2011*

**Awakening Compassion at Work: the quiet power that elevates people and organsiations** by M.C. Worline and J.E. Dutton
*Berrett-Koehler Publishers, California 2017*

**Time to Care: How to love your patients and your job** by R. Youngson
*Rebel Heart Publishers, New Zealand 2012*

# RESOURCES

If you are in distress, here are a few organisations that can help you. Some are general and some are specifically for doctors. Asking for help is one of the most protective skills we can have and is core to our wellbeing. If you need help, take this important step now to practise what you encourage your patients to do and get the help you need to be well. Most medical boards and professional associations also have resources to support you on their websites. You can also check our website, https://www.coachingfordoctors.net.au/resources/links, which we update regularly.

This book is general in nature, and while it has lots of knowledge and many useful strategies, it should not be your only resource for support.

## Australia

DRS4DRS
  https://drs4drs.com.au
  *Doctors' health advisory and referral services, offering independent, safe, supportive and confidential services.*

Hand-n-Hand Peer Support
  https://www.handnhand.org.au
  *Free, confidential peer support for health professionals in Australia and New Zealand offering emotional and wellbeing assistance, connecting through lived experience.*

Suicide Call Back Service
  https://www.suicidecallbackservice.org.au    1300 659 467
  *Suicide Call Back Service is a nationwide service providing 24/7 telephone and online counselling to people affected by suicide.*

Lifeline
  https://www.lifeline.org.au                    **13 11 14**
  *Providing all Australians experiencing emotional distress with access to 24 hour crisis support and suicide prevention services.*

Beyond Blue
https://www.beyondblue.org.au          1300 22 4636
*Information and support to help Australians achieve their best possible mental health, whatever their age and wherever they live.*

Black Dog Institute
https://www.blackdoginstitute.org.au
*Researching the early detection, prevention and treatment of common mental health disorders*

Postgraduate Medical Council of Victoria
https://www.pmcv.com.au/jmos
*Systemic and individual wellbeing support community and services for junior medical officers in Victoria*

## New Zealand

Lifeline New Zealand
https://www.lifeline.org.nz          **0800 543 354**

Suicide Crisis Helpline          0508 828 865 (0508 TAUTOKO)

## United States

Physician Support Line
https://www.physiciansupportline.com          **1 (888) 409-0141**
*Psychiatrists supporting physicians and medical students*

Suicide Prevention Lifeline
https://suicidepreventionlifeline.org          1 (800) 273-8255

## United Kingdom

Doctors in Distress
https://doctors-in-distress.org.uk
*Support groups aimed at reducing burnout and suicide in the medical profession*

Supportline
https://www.supportline.org.uk/about/about-supportline          **01708 765200**

# ABOUT THE AUTHOR

Sharee is a registered psychologist, executive coach, facilitator, and meditation teacher. She is the founder of Coaching for Doctors, Australia's first coaching practice dedicated solely to doctor development.

She has been working as a psychologist for nearly three decades, building a deep knowledge about enhancing human performance, well-being, and mental health.

She has spent the past seven years in conversation with doctors, individually and in immersion groups, seeking to understand their experience of work and their goals for their futures and the future of the health system.

She has taken to heart the findings that healthy providers of care achieve better health outcomes for patients and have more joy and satisfaction in their work. Sharee believes that by collectively raising our skills in emotional intelligence, emotional regulation, mindfulness and compassion, we will change the way we "do" healthcare for everyone's benefit.

The coaching relationship is a place of confidential reflective thinking and experiences that facilitates creativity and growth. This process fosters insight, supports change, and identifies assumptions that may be limiting progress. Coaching with Sharee is about building personal capacity for improved performance, greater wellbeing, stronger relationships and more balance.

As doctors develop their intra and interpersonal skills, they naturally behave in ways that change how healthcare is delivered. Sharee is committed to helping doctors thrive for their own benefit and that of their patients.

She initiated and codesigned the immersion doctor care program *Recalibrate* with doctors, to amplify her work with individual doctors, recognising that for people to truly thrive they need to connect with others and feel like they belong in a safe community.

Sharee is the proud mother of three amazing young people and a member of an incredible community in regional Victoria.

# CONNECT WITH ME

If you have connected with this book, I'd love to hear what has resonated with you. What have you found useful, and how have you applied it? If you'd like to know more about how you can develop your skills in taking care of yourself or connecting with others, there are many ways for us to work together.

The most impactful way is to join our signature immersion doctor care program *Recalibrate*. You can keep track of when each group is starting their work by signing up to our monthly newsletter:

https://www.coachingfordoctors.net.au
Linkedin – shareejohnson
Instagram – shareejohnsoncoaching
Facebook – Coaching for Doctors

www.ingramcontent.com/pod-product-compliance
Lightning Source LLC
Chambersburg PA
CBHW022045020426
42335CB00012B/544